Chest X-Rays for Medical Students

Chest X-Rays for Medical Students

CXRs made easy

Second Edition

Christopher Clarke
Consultant Radiologist
Nottingham University Hospitals NHS Trust
Nottingham, UK

Anthony Dux
Former Consultant Radiologist
University Hospitals of Leicester NHS Trust
Leicester, UK

WILEY Blackwell

This edition first published 2020
© 2020 John Wiley & Sons Ltd

Edition History
Wiley-Blackwell (1e, 2011)

Registered Office(s)
John Wiley & Sons, Inc., 111 River Street, Hoboken, NJ 07030, USA
John Wiley & Sons Ltd, The Atrium, Southern Gate, Chichester, West Sussex, PO19 8SQ, UK

Editorial Office
9600 Garsington Road, Oxford, OX4 2DQ, UK

For details of our global editorial offices, customer services, and more information about Wiley products visit us at www.wiley.com.

Wiley also publishes its books in a variety of electronic formats and by print-on-demand. Some content that appears in standard print versions of this book may not be available in other formats.

Library of Congress Cataloging-in-Publication Data
Names: Clarke, Christopher, 1986– author. | Dux, Anthony, author.
Title: Chest x-rays for medical students : CXRs made easy / Christopher
    Clarke, Anthony Dux.
Description: Second edition. | Hoboken, NJ : Wiley-Blackwell, 2020. |
    Includes bibliographical references and index.
Identifiers: LCCN 2019047688 (print) | LCCN 2019047689 (ebook) | ISBN
    9781119504153 (paperback) | ISBN 9781119504054 (adobe pdf) | ISBN
    9781119504122 (epub)
Subjects: MESH: Radiography, Thoracic–methods | Radiography | Thoracic
    Diseases–diagnostic imaging | Thorax–pathology | Atlas
Classification: LCC RC78 (print) | LCC RC78 (ebook) | NLM WF 17 | DDC
    616.07/572–dc23
LC record available at https://lccn.loc.gov/2019047688
LC ebook record available at https://lccn.loc.gov/2019047689

Cover Design: Wiley
Cover Image: Courtesy of Christopher Clarke

Set in 11.5/13.5pt STIXTwoText by SPi Global, Pondicherry, India
Printed and bound in Singapore by Markono Print Media Pte Ltd

10 9 8 7 6 5 4 3 2 1

Contents

Preface to the 2nd Edition

The original reason behind this book was an attempt to create a written manual of an approach to chest X-rays used in medical school teaching. Its aim was to discourage pure 'pattern recognition' as a means for identifying chest abnormalities, but instead to adopt a methodical and analytical approach which would allow an understanding of both standard and complex cases. Essentially, the method encourages an understanding of basic anatomical and pathological detail as well as the physics behind the image, whilst at all times remembering that the chest radiograph is a two-dimensional representation of a three-dimensional object.

This second edition adheres to the principles of its predecessor, whilst updating it by adding important revisions and new images as well as pathologies. We have changed and updated most of the images throughout the book with clearer annotations and higher quality images.

There is a new section specifically on nasogastric (NG) tubes, with an easy guide on correct NG tube positioning. There is new information on positioning of vascular access catheters and tubes. There are new illustrations to explain complex radiological appearances in an easy to understand way, including consolidation and the 'silhouette sign'. Clinical details have been added to the self-test questions, and there are many other additions to make this a one-stop guide to learning chest radiograph interpretation.

Our thanks, as always, to our publisher for requesting this updated second edition.

Dr Christopher Clarke

Dr Anthony Dux

Acknowledgements

We would like to thank the radiographers and staff at Nottingham University Hospitals NHS Trust and University Hospitals of Leicester NHS Trust, without whose dedication and work none of this would have been possible. We would like to thank the University of Leicester and the University of Nottingham for the use of their libraries and excellent audiovisual services. Thank you to David Heney and Stewart Peterson for their advice and encouragement, without whose support we would not have been able to complete the first edition. Special thanks to the hundreds of students who attended the focus group and lectures over the years and gave fantastic constructive feedback. Their suggestions and contributions shaped this book and were invaluable.

We would like to acknowledge our friends and colleagues who have read this text and made numerous suggestions and contributions. Thanks to Martin Davies and Karen Moore from Wiley-Blackwell for giving us the opportunity to see our work published, and to Magenta Styles for giving us the opportunity to update our work in this second edition. Finally, to all those who helped us but remain unnamed in this acknowledgement, we are very grateful.

Learning objectives checklist

*K*eep track of your learning by ticking the □ when you have covered the topic. By the end of this workbook, students should:

- □ Have a basic understanding of the principle of X-rays and how the image is produced.
- □ Have a system to use for analysing (ABCDE) and presenting chest radiographs.
- □ Know how to recognise the following on a chest radiograph:
  - □ Rotation
  - □ Adequate inspiration
  - □ Tracheal deviation
  - □ Carinal angle
  - □ Consolidation/airspace opacification
  - □ Air bronchogram
  - □ Right upper lobe collapse
  - □ Middle lobe collapse
  - □ Right lower lobe collapse
  - □ Left upper lobe collapse
  - □ Left lower lobe collapse
  - □ Complete lung collapse
  - □ Pneumonectomy
  - □ Solitary mass lesion
  - □ Multiple mass lesions
  - □ Cavitating lung lesion
  - □ Fibrosis
  - □ Pneumothorax
  - □ Tension pneumothorax
  - □ Hydropneumothorax
  - □ Pleural effusion
  - □ Pulmonary oedema
    - □ 'Bat's wing' pattern opacification
  - □ Septal lines
  - □ Asbestos-related lung disease
    - □ Benign pleural disease
    - □ Asbestosis
    - □ Mesothelioma
  - □ Dextrocardia
  - □ Cardiomegaly (enlarged heart)
  - □ Left atrial enlargement
  - □ Widened mediastinum
  - □ Hilar enlargement
  - □ Hiatus hernia
  - □ Fractures
  - □ Sclerotic and lucent bone lesions
  - □ Gas under the diaphragm (pneumoperitoneum)

☐ Subcutaneous emphysema/surgical emphysema
☐ Mastectomy
☐ Medical and surgical objects (iatrogenic)
☐ Foreign bodies
☐ Heart failure
☐ Tuberculosis (TB)

About the companion website

Don't forget to visit the companion website for this book:

www.wiley.com/go/clarke-cxr-2e

The website contains self assessment questions and answers.

Introduction
to X-rays

1 Introduction to X-rays

What are X-rays?

X-rays are a form of **ionising radiation.** Radiation is the transfer of energy in the form of particles or waves. Visible light, radio waves, and ultraviolet waves are all examples of radiation and form part of the electromagnetic spectrum. X-rays contain more energy than visible light and ultraviolet waves. In fact, X-rays have sufficient energy to cause ionisations, which is a process whereby radiation removes an outer-shell electron from an atom, hence the term ionising radiation. In this way, ionising radiation is able to cause changes on a molecular level in biologically important molecules (e.g. DNA).

Uses of ionising radiation include conventional plain radiographs (often simply referred to as X-rays), fluoroscopy, computed tomography (CT), nuclear medicine, and positron emission tomography (PET).

How are X-rays produced?

X-rays are produced by focusing a high-energy beam of electrons onto a metal target (e.g. tungsten) (Figure 1.1). The electrons hit the metal target and some will have enough energy to knock out another electron from the inner shell of one of the metal atoms. As a result, electrons from higher energy levels then fill up this vacancy and X-rays are emitted in the process. Producing X-rays this way is extremely inefficient (~0.1%), so most of the energy is wasted as heat. For this reason, X-ray tubes need to have advanced cooling mechanisms. The X-rays produced then pass through the patient and onto a detector mechanism which produces an image.

Chest X-rays for Medical Students: CXRs Made Easy, Second Edition.
Christopher Clarke and Anthony Dux.
© 2020 John Wiley & Sons Ltd. Published 2020 by John Wiley & Sons Ltd.
Companion website: www.wiley.com/go/clarke-cxr-2e

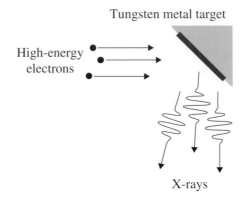

Figure 1.1 X-ray production.

How do X-rays make an image?

X-rays can either pass through the body or be absorbed by tissues. While passing through a patient, the X-ray beam is absorbed in proportion to the cube of the atomic number of the various tissues through which it passes. A simple way to think about this is to remember that the denser a structure is, the more X-rays are absorbed.

Any X-rays that are not absorbed are detected by the detector plate. By convention, the greater the number of X-rays hitting a detector, the blacker the image will be. Therefore, the less dense a material is, the more X-rays get through and the blacker the image will be. Conversely the more dense a material is, the more X-rays are absorbed and the image appears whiter. In summary, materials of high density (e.g. bone) appear whiter than materials of low density (e.g. air).

It is also important to remember the following points:

1. The resulting image on the detector is a **two-dimensional (2D) representation of a three-dimensional (3D) structure.** Remember you are usually not seeing a single structure but the combined density of all the structures that an X-ray beam passes through. For example, when looking at a rib on a chest X-ray, you are also looking at the overlying subcutaneous fat, lung, and chest wall musculature. It is also important to note that the shade of grey is not only determined by the density of tissue, but also its thickness. Thicker tissues absorb more X-rays and turn the radiograph whiter.
2. **Structures can only be seen if there is sufficient contrast with surrounding tissues.** Contrast is the difference in absorption between one tissue and another.

The five densities on an X-ray

All images are comprised of a combination of the following five densities (Figure 1.2).

How are X-ray images (radiographs) stored?

Almost all hospitals use a computer-based digital radiograph storage system for storing X-ray images. This system is known as **P**icture **A**rchiving and **C**ommunication **S**ystem (**PACS**). Doctors and other healthcare professionals

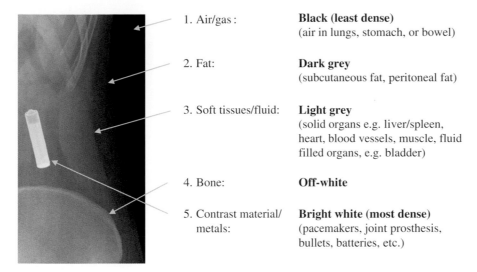

1. Air/gas :	**Black (least dense)** (air in lungs, stomach, or bowel)
2. Fat:	**Dark grey** (subcutaneous fat, peritoneal fat)
3. Soft tissues/fluid:	**Light grey** (solid organs e.g. liver/spleen, heart, blood vessels, muscle, fluid filled organs, e.g. bladder)
4. Bone:	**Off-white**
5. Contrast material/ metals:	**Bright white (most dense)** (pacemakers, joint prosthesis, bullets, batteries, etc.)

Figure 1.2 The spectrum of tissues of different densities as seen on a plain radiograph. This example is of a patient who swallowed a battery.

are able to view the images (radiographs) on a computer screen, making it easy to manipulate the image (e.g. changing the contrast, zooming in/out, etc.) and view images anywhere within the hospital.

Hazards and precautions

Ionising radiation hazards

As mentioned earlier, ionising radiation has the potential to damage cells. Actively dividing cells are particularly sensitive to radiation (e.g. bone marrow and gonads). Damage takes many forms, including cell death, mitotic inhibition, and chromosome/genetic damage leading to mutations.

The radiation dose from a chest X-ray is relatively low and equivalent to approximately three days of background radiation (Table 1.1). Having said this, patients often receive multiple X-rays during a hospital visit and over their life-time; therefore, the cumulative dose increases over time. It is therefore important to optimise the radiation dose to as low as reasonably achievable, while still obtaining an image of good diagnostic quality.

The safety of patients and the use of ionising radiation for medical exposures are subject to specific legislation in the UK – the Ionising Radiation (Medical Exposure) Regulations or IRMER.

The Ionising Radiation (Medical Exposure) Regulations (IRMER)

IRMER is UK legislation and lays down the basic measures for radiation protection for patients. It refers to three main people involved in protecting the patient:

1. The **Referrer** – a qualified doctor or other accredited health professional (e.g. emergency nurse practitioner) requesting the exposure.
   Must provide adequate and relevant clinical information to enable the practitioner to justify the exposure.

Table 1.1 Comparison of typical doses from sources of exposure.

Source of exposure	Typical effective radiation dose (mSv)	Equivalent period of natural background radiation[1]	Lifetime additional risk of fatal cancer per exposure
Limb and joint radiograph (except hip)	<0.01	<1.5 days	1 in a few million
Chest radiograph	0.02	3 days	1 in a million
Transatlantic flight	0.08	12 days	1 in 200 000
Abdominal radiograph	0.5	3 months	1 in 30 000
CT head	2	1 year	1 in 10 000
CT chest	8	3.6 years	1 in 2500

1 UK average = 2.7 mSv per year
Data taken from 'Patient dose information: guidance by Public Health England', published 4 September 2008 and 'Ionising radiation: dose comparisons by Public Health England', published 18 March 2011.

2. The **Practitioner** – usually a radiologist, who justifies the exposure.
   Decides on the appropriate imaging and justifies any exposure to radiation on a case-by-case basis. The potential benefit must outweigh the risk to the patient. (For example, a CT head scan on a one year-old adds a 1/500 lifetime risk of cancer and increases the risk of cataract formation. The benefit of this scan must therefore outweigh these risks to the child.)
3. The **Operator** – usually a radiographer, who performs practical aspects.
   Ensures that the above two stages have been completed appropriately and keeps all justifiable exposure as low as reasonably possible by:
   i. minimising the number of radiographs taken;
   ii. focusing the X-ray beam on the area of interest;
   iii. minimising the use of mobile X-ray;
   iv. keeping exposure as low as reasonably achievable.

In women of reproductive age

- Minimise radiation exposure of the abdomen and pelvis.
- Ask any woman of reproductive age if they could be pregnant and avoid radiation exposure to them. The most critical periods are the first and second trimester. From the standpoint of future development, the foetus is considered to be most radiosensitive during the second trimester when foetal organogenesis is taking place. X-rays of the abdomen and pelvis should be delayed, if possible, to a time when foetal sensitivity is reduced (i.e. post 24 weeks' gestation, or ideally until the baby is born).
- Exposure to remote areas (chest, skull, and limbs) may be undertaken with minimal fetal exposure at any time during pregnancy.

2 Chest X-ray views

PA erect chest X-ray

The standard view is a **PA (posterior–anterior) erect chest X-ray (CXR) (Figure 2.1).** All CXRs are taken PA erect unless otherwise stated. As a general rule, assume that a chest radiograph is taken PA erect unless it has the words **AP** or **supine** written on it.

The patient stands upright, facing the X-ray detector with their anterior chest wall pressed against it. The X-ray tube is placed approximately 6 ft. behind the patient so the X-rays pass through the patient in the posterior–anterior direction. The patient is asked to take a deep breath and hold it during the X-ray to ensure there is adequate inspiration and no breathing movement (which could make the image blurry).

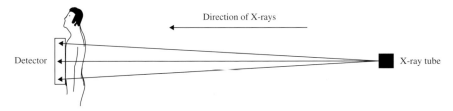

Figure 2.1 Posterior–anterior (PA) erect chest X-ray.

Reasons for performing CXRs in the PA direction are:

1. **Accurate assessment of the cardiac size due to minimal magnification.**
2. **The scapulae can be rotated out of the way.**

Reasons for performing the radiograph erect are:

1. **Gas passes upwards:** pneumothorax and free gas underneath the diaphragm are more easily diagnosed.
2. **Fluid passes downwards:** pleural effusion is more easily diagnosed.

Chest X-rays for Medical Students: CXRs Made Easy, Second Edition.
Christopher Clarke and Anthony Dux.
© 2020 John Wiley & Sons Ltd. Published 2020 by John Wiley & Sons Ltd.
Companion website: www.wiley.com/go/clarke-cxr-2e

3. **Physiological representation of blood vessels and lungs:** if it were taken in the supine position (on their back), the mediastinal veins and upper lobe vessels may be more distended than normal, leading to misinterpretation.

Other views

- **AP (anterior–posterior)/supine CXR** is performed when the patient is too ill to stand (e.g. in the intensive care unit or emergency department resuscitation). The X-ray tube is placed in front of the patient and the X-rays pass in the anterior–posterior direction. The major disadvantage of AP/supine radiographs when compared with PA radiographs is that the mediastinum and cardiac size will appear wider due to venous distension and magnification. Therefore, you should not comment on the cardiac or mediastinal enlargement on an AP/supine radiograph.
- **Lateral CXR** is an X-ray taken from the side of the patient and may be used to give further views of the lungs and heart, and more detail on the anatomical location of lesions. It is rarely performed nowadays as almost all lesions on lateral radiographs can also be seen on frontal (PA or AP/ supine) radiographs, and if more information on the location of lesions is required, then a CT scan of the chest is more precise. For these reasons we have decided not to cover lateral radiographs in this book.

3 Radiograph quality

The quality of chest radiographs can vary widely. Before you think about the possible abnormalities on a chest radiograph, you must first assess the technical quality to ensure the image is adequate. The main questions to ask yourself are:

1. Has everything been included on the radiograph?
2. Is the radiograph rotated?
3. Is the inspiration adequate?

> **Note:** You may find that some doctors will also want you to comment on whether the exposure of the radiograph is adequate. However, this is often not necessary, as images that are over- or under-exposed are terminated almost straight away by the radiographer and taken again. Also, with a computer X-ray viewer, you can change the contrast and brightness with the mouse to compensate for poor exposure.

Inclusion

The entire anatomy should be included from the lung apices to the both costophrenic angles (Figure 3.1).

- The lung apices (1) should be included at the top of the radiograph.
- The lateral aspects of the ribcage (2) should be seen on either side of the radiograph.
- The left and right costophrenic angles (3) should be included at the bottom of the radiograph.

Chest X-rays for Medical Students: CXRs Made Easy, Second Edition.
Christopher Clarke and Anthony Dux.
© 2020 John Wiley & Sons Ltd. Published 2020 by John Wiley & Sons Ltd.
Companion website: www.wiley.com/go/clarke-cxr-2e

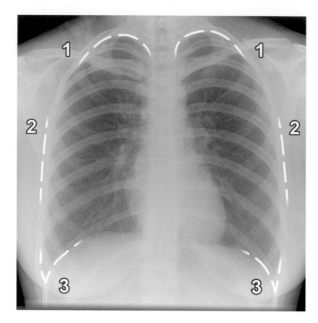

Figure 3.1 A normal chest radiograph showing the lung apices (1), lateral aspects of the ribcage (2), and both costophrenic angles (3) marked with dashed white lines.

Rotation

It is important to assess rotation as a rotated radiograph can make the heart and mediastinum look larger or smaller than they actually are and may obscure pathology.

Look at the spinous processes of the upper thoracic vertebrae. If the patient is not rotated they should lie midway between the medial ends of the clavicles. If the patient is rotated the spinous processes of the upper thoracic vertebrae will not lie midway between the medial ends of the clavicles but will be deviated to either the left or right side.

- **Patient is rotated to the left:** the medial ends of the clavicles will be deviated to the left (patient's left) of the spinous processes of the upper thoracic vertebrae.
- **Patient is rotated to the right:** the medial ends of the clavicles will be deviated to the right (patient's right) of the spinous processes of the upper thoracic vertebrae.

Note: This rule works for both PA and AP films.

Non-rotated example: Figure 3.2

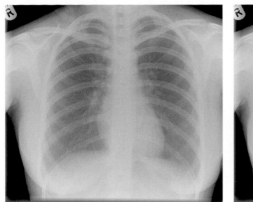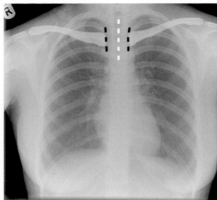

Figure 3.2 Non-rotated chest radiograph. The clavicles are yellow and the medial ends of the clavicles are marked with a black dotted line. The position of the spinous processes of the upper thoracic vertebrae are shown with a white dotted line. The spinous processes lie midway between the medial ends of the clavicles, therefore this radiograph is not rotated.

Rotated example: Figure 3.3

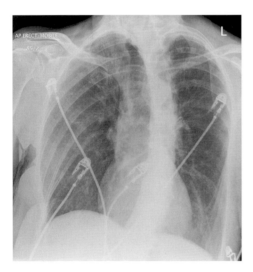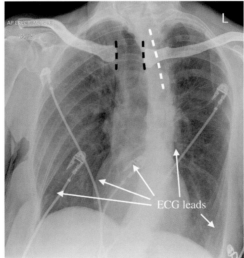

Figure 3.3 Chest radiograph of a patient rotated to the right. The clavicles are marked in yellow and the medial ends of the clavicles are marked with a black dotted line. The position of the spinous processes of the upper thoracic vertebrae are shown with a white dotted line. The medial ends of the clavicles are deviated to the right of the spinous processes, therefore this radiograph is rotated to the right.

Inspiration

Adequate inspiration is important as if the inspiration is too shallow the heart may appear falsely enlarged, giving the false appearance of cardiomegaly. Also, if the lungs are not adequately inflated, the vessels at the lung bases can look more prominent and give the false appearance of consolidation or collapse.

Inspiration is considered adequate if the hemidiaphragms lie at or below the level of the anterior part of the 6th ribs. Alternatively, if the posterior part of the 8th or 9th ribs are clearly visible in the lung fields, this also indicates adequate inspiration.

Example of adequate inspiration: Figure 3.4

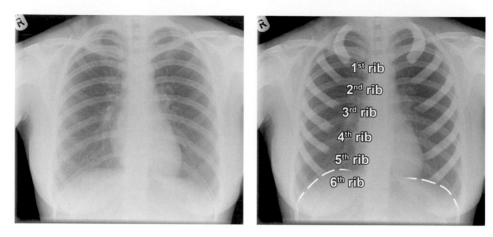

Figure 3.4 Chest radiograph with adequate inspiration. The right radiograph shows the anterior parts of the 1st to 6th ribs marked in yellow and the left and right hemidiaphragm are marked with dashed white lines.

If the lungs are under-inflated, then there will be five or fewer anterior ribs (or seven or fewer posterior ribs) visible overlying the lung fields.

Example of inadequate inspiration: Figure 3.5

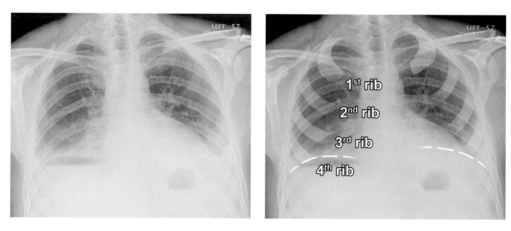

Figure 3.5 Chest radiograph with inadequate inspiration. Notice how the lung volumes are smaller when compared to the previous figure (Figure 3.4). There is the false appearance of cardiomegaly. The anterior parts of the 1st to 4th ribs are marked in yellow and the left and right hemidiaphragm are marked with dashed white lines. (In this example, you can also see gas under the right hemidiaphragm in keeping with pneumoperitoneum.)

4

Normal anatomy on a PA chest X-ray

The following normal chest radiographs show the normal chest anatomy.

Right and left

Remember, as you look at a chest radiograph, the left side of the image is the patient's right side, and the right side of the image is the patient's left side (Figure 4.1). Always describe findings according to the patient's side.

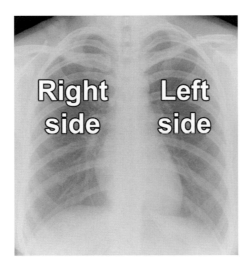

Figure 4.1 A normal chest radiograph showing the left and right side.

> **Note:** A good way to remember this is to imagine that the patient is always facing towards you. This is true for both PA and AP films.

Chest X-rays for Medical Students: CXRs Made Easy, Second Edition.
Christopher Clarke and Anthony Dux.
© 2020 John Wiley & Sons Ltd. Published 2020 by John Wiley & Sons Ltd.
Companion website: www.wiley.com/go/clarke-cxr-2e

Lung zones

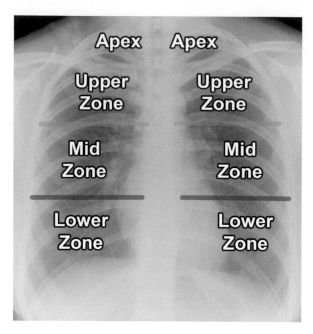

Figure 4.2 A normal chest radiograph demonstrating lung zone anatomy.

Knowing the lung zones is useful when describing where an abnormality is located (Figure 4.2). If you are unable to work out the exact lobe a lesion is located in, then describe the zone.

The mediastinum

The mediastinum, marked in orange, is the central part of the thoracic cavity (Figure 4.3).

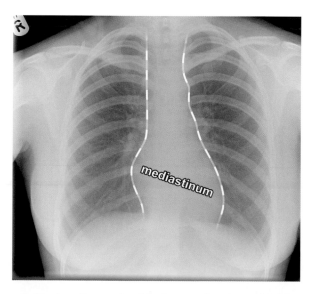

Figure 4.3 A normal chest radiograph with the mediastinum highlighted in orange.

It contains the heart, the great vessels, oesophagus, trachea, phrenic nerve, vagus nerve, sympathetic chain, thoracic duct, thymus, and central lymph nodes.

Normal pulmonary vasculature

The normal lung vascular pattern has the following features (Figure 4.4):

- **arteries** and **veins** branching from the mediastinum into the lungs;
- the upper lobe vessels have a smaller diameter than the lower lobe vessels on an erect chest radiograph.

The main pulmonary vascular markings of a normal chest radiograph are highlighted in red. The white dotted line indicates the level at which the pulmonary vessels enter and leave the lungs. As you can see, it is normal for the left pulmonary vasculature to be slightly higher than the right. Notice how the vessels branching upwards (the vessels above the white dotted line) are generally smaller than the vessels branching downwards (the vessels below the white dotted line). This is due to the effect of gravity.

As the pulmonary vasculature gets further away from the mediastinum, the vessels get smaller. **Lung markings** refers to all these small blood vessels seen on a chest radiograph. If each lung is divided into thirds, from the inside to the outside, you can appreciate how the normal lung markings change (Figure 4.5):

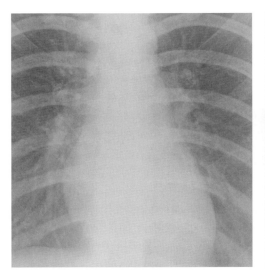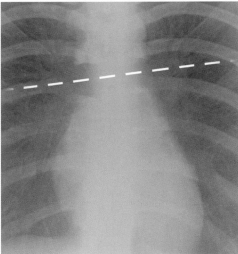

Figure 4.4 A normal chest radiograph with the pulmonary vascular markings in red.

Note: The opposite can occur in pulmonary venous hypertension, i.e. the vessels branching upwards become larger than the vessels branching downwards.

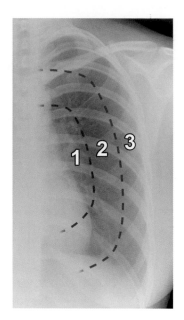

Figure 4.5 Left half of a chest radiograph demonstrating changes in lung markings from medial to lateral.

Centre	**1.** Clearly defined vessels and bronchial branches ...	**2.** ... become smaller and more difficult to see.	**3.** Fine pattern of branching lines with no easily defined vessels or airspaces.	Pleura

Inside ⟶ **Outside**

General anatomy

General anatomy 1: Figure 4.6

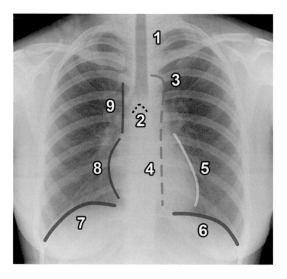

1. **Trachea** (light blue)
2. **Carina – spinal level T5** (black dotted line)
3. **Aortic arch/knuckle** (green)
4. **Descending thoracic aorta** (green dashed line)
5. **Left heart border** (yellow)
6. **Left hemidiaphragm** (pink)
7. **Right hemidiaphragm** (purple)
8. **Right heart border** (red)
9. **Superior vena cava** (blue)

Figure 4.6 A chest radiograph demonstrating normal anatomy.

The left ventricle forms the left heart border and the right atrium forms the right heart border. Neither the left atrium nor the right ventricle are visible on the normal chest radiograph. This is because the right ventricle lies anteriorly and the left atrium lies posteriorly, and they therefore have no definable border on a frontal chest X-ray.

General anatomy 2: Figure 4.7

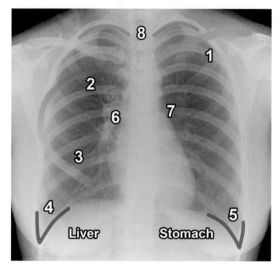

Figure 4.7 A chest radiograph demonstrating normal anatomy.

1. **Clavicle** (green)
2. **5th rib – posterior aspect** (red)
3. **5th rib – anterior aspect** (yellow)
4. **Right costophrenic angle** (purple)
5. **Left costophrenic angle** (pink)
6. **Right hilum** (containing the right hilar lymph nodes) (light blue)
7. **Left hilum** (containing the left hilar lymph nodes) (blue)
8. **Lung apex** (*pl.* apices) (orange)

The hilar regions (Figure 4.7) are where the pulmonary arteries, pulmonary veins, and main bronchi enter the lungs from the mediastinum. There are lots of small lymph nodes around these vessels called the hilar lymph nodes. If these hilar lymph nodes are enlarged, then they may be visible on visible on a chest radiograph. Both the left and right hilar regions contain the same structures; however, they are not symmetrical, the left is usually slightly higher than the right.

Bronchial and lobar anatomy: Figure 4.8

1. **Trachea**
2. **Carina** – spinal level T5
3. **Left main bronchus**
4. **Right main bronchus**
5. **Left upper lobe bronchus**
6. **Left lower lobe bronchus**
7. **Right upper lobe bronchus**
8. **Intermediate bronchus**
9. **Middle lobe bronchus**
10. **Right lower lobe bronchus**

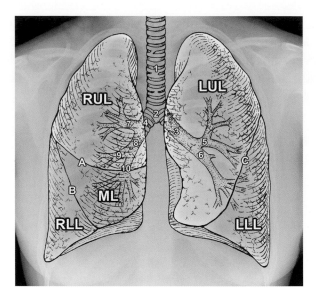

Figure 4.8 A normal chest radiograph showing the bronchial and lobar anatomy.

A. Horizontal fissure
B. Right oblique fissure
C. Left oblique fissure

RUL. **Right upper lobe** (pink)
ML. **Middle lobe** (purple)
RLL. **Right lower lobe** (blue)
LUL. **Left upper lobe** (pink)
LLL. **Left lower lobe** (blue)

The trachea (1) divides at the carina (2) to give off the left main bronchus (3) and right main bronchus (4).

The left main bronchus splits into the upper lobe bronchus (5) and lower lobe bronchus (6).

The right main bronchus gives off the upper lobe bronchus (7) and continues inferiorly as the intermediate bronchus (8), which subsequently bifurcates into the middle lobe bronchus (9) and lower lobe bronchus (10).

The right upper lobe (RUL) is separated from the middle lobe (ML) by the **horizontal fissure** (A). The middle lobe is separated from the right lower lobe (RLL) by the **right oblique fissure** (B). The left upper lobe (LUL) is separated from the left lower lobe (LLL) by the **left oblique fissure** (C).

There are two upper and two lower lobes, but only one middle lobe which is situated in the right lung. As the middle lobe is only found on the right side there is no need to describe it as 'right middle lobe'. You should simply call it the 'middle lobe'.

The part of the left upper lobe which lies adjacent to the left ventricle (the lower half of the left upper lobe) is called the **lingula.**

5

Presenting a chest radiograph

You should present a chest radiograph in a systematic way to ensure you review all areas and do not miss anything important. This is how you should present.

1. Give the **type** of radiograph and **projection**. 2. Give the patient's name. 3. Give the date the X-ray was taken.	*E.g. 'This is a PA **chest radiograph** of John Smith, taken on the 1st of January.'*
4. Briefly assess the radiograph quality to ensure it is adequate. 5. Run through the ABCDE of chest X-rays.	See sections on 'Radiograph quality' and 'ABCDE of chest X-rays'.
6. Give a short summary at the end.	

Always remember to give a detailed description of what you see. A good way to think about this is to imagine you are describing the radiograph to a colleague over the phone. If you see something abnormal you must say **where it is anatomically** and **what it looks like.**

There are 18 examples of describing a CXR in *www.wiley.com/go/clarke-cxr-2e*.

Example of presenting a normal chest X-ray

'This is a PA chest radiograph of John Smith, taken on the 1st of January.'

'The radiograph is not rotated and there is adequate inspiration.'

A: 'The trachea is central.'

B: 'The lungs are uniformly expanded and the lung fields are clear.'

Chest X-rays for Medical Students: CXRs Made Easy, Second Edition.
Christopher Clarke and Anthony Dux.
© 2020 John Wiley & Sons Ltd. Published 2020 by John Wiley & Sons Ltd.
Companion website: www.wiley.com/go/clarke-cxr-2e

C: 'The heart size is normal. There is no mediastinal shift. The mediastinal contours and hila appear normal.'

D: 'There is no fracture or bone abnormality.'

E: 'There is no evidence of gas under the diaphragm, subcutaneous emphysema, or any foreign body.'

'In summary, this is a normal chest radiograph.'

The ABCDE of chest X-rays

It is important to use a systematic approach when looking at a chest radiograph. The following ABCDE approach is easy to remember, so when it comes to your exams and you have a moment of panic after being asked to talk about a chest X-ray, you can stick to these basics even if you don't have a clue what's going on!

A is for Airway:

- Look at the trachea and right and left main bronchi.

B is for Breathing:

- Look to see if the lungs are uniformly expanded and compare the lung fields.
- Look around the edges of each lung.
- Look at the costophrenic angles and the four silhouettes.

C is for Circulation:

- Look at the cardiac size.
- Look at the great vessels (pulmonary vessels and aorta).
- Look at the mediastinum and hila.

D is for Disability:

- Look for a fracture, especially of the ribs or shoulder girdle.

E is for Everything else (review areas):

- Look for gas under the diaphragm.
- Look for surgical emphysema.
- Look for both breast shadows.
- Look for foreign bodies and medical interventions.

Chest X-rays for Medical Students: CXRs Made Easy, Second Edition.
Christopher Clarke and Anthony Dux.
© 2020 John Wiley & Sons Ltd. Published 2020 by John Wiley & Sons Ltd.
Companion website: www.wiley.com/go/clarke-cxr-2e

6

A – Airway

How to review the airway

Start at the top and follow the **trachea (1)** inferiorly. It should lie in the midline. It divides at the **carina (2)** to give off the **right main bronchus (3)** and **left main bronchus (4)** (Figure 6.1). On a normal radiograph you will often not be able to visualise the more distal airway branches.

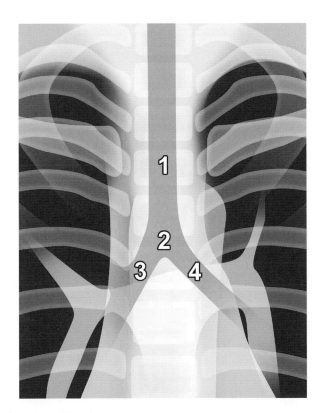

Figure 6.1 The airways of the lung.

Chest X-rays for Medical Students: CXRs Made Easy, Second Edition.
Christopher Clarke and Anthony Dux.
© 2020 John Wiley & Sons Ltd. Published 2020 by John Wiley & Sons Ltd.
Companion website: www.wiley.com/go/clarke-cxr-2e

What to look for

- Tracheal deviation   p. 24
- Carinal angle   p. 25

Tracheal deviation

The trachea is considered to be deviated if a portion, anywhere along its length, is completely to the left or right of the midline (the midline being the centre of the vertebral column as indicated by the spinous processes).

If you suspect that the trachea is deviated, look for a possible cause.

> **Note:** Be sure to check that the radiograph is not rotated, as a rotated radiograph can give the impression of tracheal deviation when the trachea is actually central.

- **Deviated towards diseased side** (conditions that pull the trachea):
  - *lung collapse;*
  - *pneumonectomy* (removal of a lung) or lobectomy (removal of just one lobe);
  - unilateral fibrosis;
  - agenesis of lung (also called lung aplasia – complete absence of a whole lung and its bronchus).
- **Deviated away from diseased side** (conditions that push the trachea):
  - *tension pneumothorax;*
  - *massive pleural effusion;*
  - mediastinal masses;
  - para-tracheal masses.

The most common causes of tracheal deviation are shown in **bold italic**.

Most other processes (consolidation, non-tension pneumothorax, etc.) have little effect on tracheal deviation.

Example: Figure 6.2

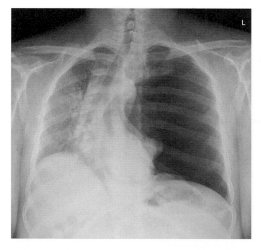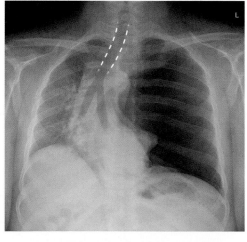

Figure 6.2 The trachea is deviated to the right of the midline. This is due to a left-sided tension pneumothorax 'pushing' the trachea away. The trachea is outlined with a white dotted line and shown in blue.

Carinal angle

The carinal angle is the **angle between** the **right main bronchus** and the **left main bronchus.** Normally the angle is between 40° and 100° (Figure 6.3). An **increase** in the **carinal angle** is an **indirect sign of pathology** in the heart, mediastinum, or lungs; therefore, if the carinal angle is greater than 100°, look for a pathology that could be causing this (Figure 6.4).

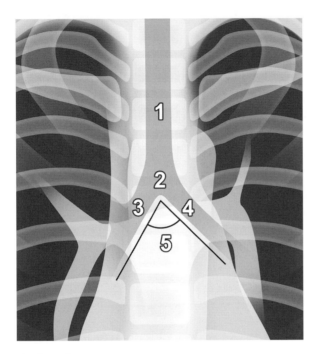

Figure 6.3 The carinal angle.

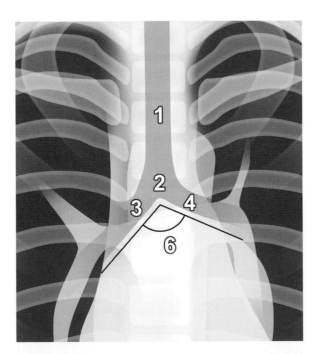

Figure 6.4 The carinal angle is widened, which could indicate pathology.

It increases if there is something pushing up from beneath the carina or if there is something pulling from above the right or left main bronchus.

1. **Trachea**
2. **Carina**
3. **Left main bronchus**
4. **Right main bronchus**
5. **Carinal angle**
6. **Widened carinal angle**

A widened carinal angle could indicate:

- **a sub-carinal mass** (i.e. a mass below the carina, e.g. bronchial carcinoma, large hiatus hernia);
- **left atrial enlargement, cardiomegaly,** or a **pericardial effusion;**
- **right or left upper lobe collapse** (pulling the main bronchus upwards).

7

B – Breathing

How to review the lungs

A general rule is that **black = air** and **white = no air.** There are five main areas to look at.

1. Are the lungs **uniformly expanded?**
2. **Compare the lung fields** and look for white areas (opacities):
   - compare left apex with right apex;
   - compare left upper zone with right upper zone;
   - compare left mid zone with the right mid zone;
   - compare the left lower zone with the right lower zone.
3. **Look around the edges of each lung.**
4. **Look at the costophrenic angles.**
5. **Look for the following four silhouettes (outlines) (Figure 7.1):**

   i. **Right heart border.** Loss of definition of the right heart border silhouette indicates a loss of air in the middle lobe (due to collapse or consolidation).
   ii. **Left heart border.** Loss of definition of the left heart border silhouette indicates a loss of air in the lingula (part of the left upper lobe).
   iii. **Right hemidiaphragm.** Loss of definition of the right hemidiaphragmatic silhouette indicates a loss of air in the right lower lobe (due to collapse or consolidation), or that there is something between the diaphragm and the right lower lobe (e.g. pleural fluid).
   iv. **Left hemidiaphragm.** Loss of definition of the left hemidiaphragmatic silhouette indicates a loss of air in the left lower lobe (due to collapse or consolidation), or that there is something between the diaphragm and the left lower lobe (e.g. pleural fluid).

Chest X-rays for Medical Students: CXRs Made Easy, Second Edition.
Christopher Clarke and Anthony Dux.
© 2020 John Wiley & Sons Ltd. Published 2020 by John Wiley & Sons Ltd.
Companion website: www.wiley.com/go/clarke-cxr-2e

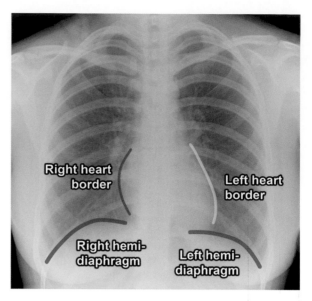

Figure 7.1 The four silhouettes. The right heart border (red), left heart border (yellow), right hemidiaphragm (purple), and left hemidiaphragm (pink).

Note: It is normal to see all four silhouettes as there should be air in the lobes adjacent to each these four areas. If there is an opacity in the lobe adjacent to one of these areas (e.g. consolidation or collapse), then the crisp silhouette is lost and this is called the '**silhouette sign**' (Figure 7.2). Because the 'silhouette sign' refers to the loss of one of the above silhouettes, it may be more accurate to call it the 'loss of silhouette sign' or 'loss of outline sign'.

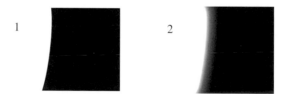

Figure 7.2 Diagrammatic representation of the silhouette sign. Image 1 (left) shows a normal crisp silhouette. Image 2 (right) shows the 'silhouette sign'. As you can see the 'silhouette sign' refers to loss of definition/blurring of the normal crisp silhouette.

What to look for

Chest X-rays do not show many specific diseases (e.g. pneumonia, primary lung malignancy, etc.), only signs of pathology, which can give a clue to the underlying disease process. The following are a list of pathologies and signs that you should know.

Consolidation/airspace opacification

Consolidation (also known as airspace opacification) is the **replacement of alveolar air** by **fluid, cells, pus,** or **other material (Figure 7.3). Pneumonia** is by far the most common cause of consolidation. It is also sometimes seen in primary TB.

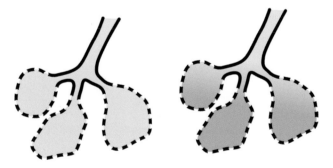

Figure 7.3 Diagrammatic representation of three normal alveoli (left image) and consolidation (green) within the three alveoli (right image).

Features of consolidation on a chest radiograph

- **Heterogenous or patchy opacification:** the opacification is non-uniform and the border is not well demarcated (it sometimes looks fluffy).
- **Lobar or segmental distribution:** the opacification usually corresponds anatomically to a lobe or lung segment.
- **Air bronchogram** (see p. 31): the presence of an air bronchogram would confirm that the density (fluid/pus) was in the alveoli and not the larger

airways. Bronchial breathing on auscultation is the clinical sign of an air bronchogram.

- **No loss of lung volume:** lung volumes may actually increase in the early stages of consolidation. In later stages there can be a small loss of lung volume due to secretions obstructing airways; however, as a general rule, there is no significant loss of lung volume in consolidation.

> **Note:** Remember the clinical history. In the presence of a temperature and signs of infection, consolidation is by far the most likely abnormality. Also compare with previous radiographs – the presence of a similar abnormality on a previous radiograph should lead you to suspect fibrosis rather than consolidation.

Example 1: Figure 7.4

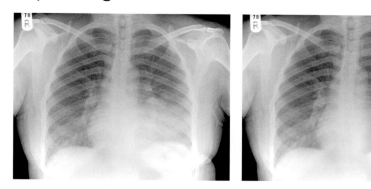

Figure 7.4 Consolidation in the lingula (green). There is heterogenous airspace opacification in the left lower zone and no loss of lung volume. The left hemidiaphragm can be clearly seen, however the left heart border is poorly defined (silhouette sign); therefore, the pathology is in the lung adjacent to the left heart border, i.e. the lingula of the left upper lobe.

Example 2: Figure 7.5

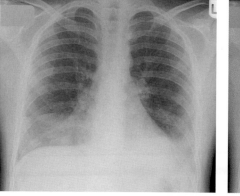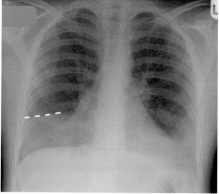

Figure 7.5 Consolidation (green) in the middle lobe and left lower lobe. There is heterogenous airspace opacification in the right and left lower zones and no loss of lung volume. We know the consolidation on the right side is in the middle lobe as there is loss of definition of the right heart border (silhouette sign) and the superior border is the horizontal fissure (marked with a white dashed line). We know the consolidation on the left side is in the left lower lobe as there is loss of definition of the left hemidiaphragm (silhouette sign), yet the left heart border is still clearly visible.

Example 3: Figure 7.6

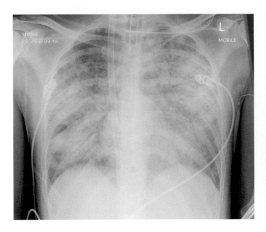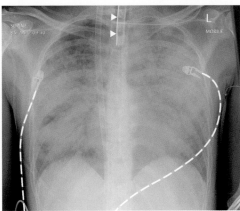

Figure 7.6 Consolidation (green) in both lungs with moderate sparing of the right upper zone (which appears darker than the rest). There is heterogenous airspace opacification, no loss of lung volume, and air bronchograms seen in both lungs. You can also see an endotracheal tube (white arrowheads), ECG leads (white dashed lines), nasogastric tube in situ, and other overlying tubing.

Air bronchogram

An air bronchogram is the **radiographic appearance** of an **air-filled bronchus** that is surrounded by **fluid-filled** or **solid alveoli.**

- It can appear when there is **consolidation** (e.g. pneumonia) or **pulmonary oedema** in the surrounding alveoli.
- Sometimes it is a good prognostic sign as it shows that secretions are able to exit from the consolidated region via the bronchus.

Note: The air bronchogram is the radiological equivalent of bronchial breathing on clinical examination.

Example 1: Figure 7.7

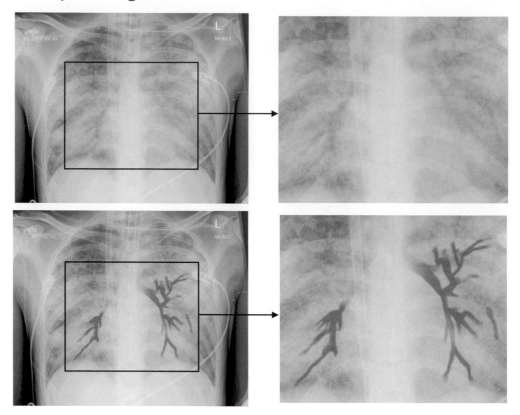

Figure 7.7 This is the same radiograph as Figure 7.6 and is a good example of an air bronchogram caused by severe bilateral consolidation. The air bronchogram is marked in grey on the inferior radiograph. You can also see an endotracheal tube, ECG leads, nasogastric tube in situ, and other overlying tubing.

Collapse (atelectasis) overview

Collapse is **failure of all or part of the lung to expand** due to **loss of air in the alveoli.**

- **Lobar collapse** refers to collapse of a particular lobe of the lung.
- **Lung collapse** refers to collapse of a whole lung.

General features of collapse on a chest radiograph include:

- An increase in **density**, representing lung devoid of air (whiteness).
- Signs indicating **decreased lung volume**, such as:
  - displacement of mediastinum/trachea towards the collapsed lung;
  - elevation of the hemidiaphragm;
  - compensatory over-inflation of adjacent lobes or opposite lung.

Note: When looking at a white lung, it is important to be thorough in looking for the possible features of collapse since the presence of collapse indicates possible serious pathology. Collapse is commonly found with consolidation (consolidation causing collapse). If this is so, it is referred to as collapse-consolidation.

Causes of collapse include:

- **Consolidation** (e.g. pneumonia).
- **Bronchial obstruction** by:
  - endobronchial tumour (a tumour invading one of the bronchi);
  - mucus plugging of major airways (asthma);
  - other tumours, lymphadenopathy, or an aneurysm compressing the bronchi causing bronchial distortion;
  - inhaled foreign body (e.g. peanut);
  - iatrogenic (endotracheal tube inserted too far).
- **External pulmonary compression** (**pleural effusion/collection** or **mass**).
- Abnormalities of surfactant production (commonly occur with oxygen toxicity and acute respiratory distress syndrome).
- Inflammatory aetiology (e.g. tuberculosis or fungal infection).
- Lung fibrosis.

Specific signs of collapse of individual lobes are shown on the following pages.

Right upper lobe collapse

The right upper lobe collapses upwards.

Features of right upper lobe collapse on a chest radiograph: Figure 7.8

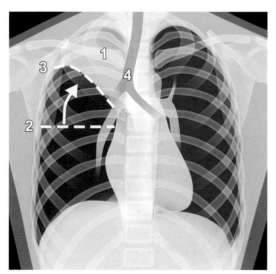

Figure 7.8 Diagrammatic representation of right upper lobe collapse. Increased density in the right upper zone (1), normal position of horizontal fissure (2), horizontal fissure displaced upwards (3), tracheal deviation to the right (4).

- Increased density in right upper zone.
- Horizontal fissure displaced upwards (pulled up by collapsed lobe).
- Loss of definition of right upper mediastinal margins.
- Elevation of right hilum (pulled up by collapsed lobe).

- Right tracheal deviation (collapsed lobe pulls trachea).
- The rest of the right lung looks blacker than the left lung (the middle lobe and right lower lobe over-inflate to compensate for the reduced volume in the hemithorax caused by the collapsed right upper lobe).

Example: Figure 7.9

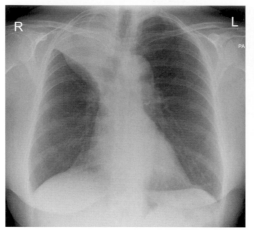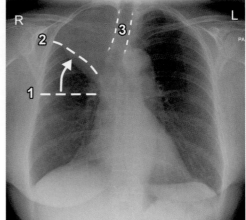

Figure 7.9 Right upper lobe collapse. There is increased opacification in the right upper zone (blue) with loss of definition of the upper right mediastinal margin. The position of the horizontal fissure in a normal lung is shown with a white dotted line (1); however, in this case the horizontal fissure has been pulled upwards (2). The volume loss from the collapsed right upper lobe has pulled the trachea to the right side (3).

Middle lobe collapse

The middle lobe collapses inwards (medially).

Features of middle lobe collapse on a chest radiograph: Figure 7.10

- Increased density in right mid-zone.
- **Loss of definition of the right heart border** (the collapsed lobe lies against the right heart border making it indistinct).
- Horizontal fissure displaced downwards (pulled down by collapsed lobe).
- The rest of the right lung looks blacker than the left lung (the right upper lobe and right lower lobe over-inflate to compensate for the reduced volume in the hemithorax caused by the collapsed lobe).

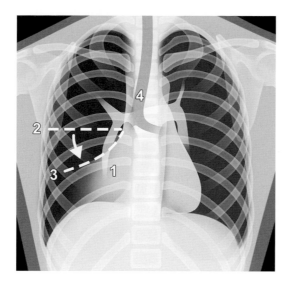

Figure 7.10 Diagrammatic representation of middle lobe collapse. Increased density in the right mid zone (1) with loss of the right heart border silhouette, normal position of horizontal fissure (2), horizontal fissure displaced downwards (3), tracheal deviation to the right (4).

Example: Figure 7.11

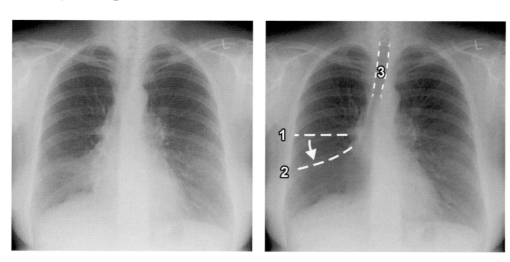

Figure 7.11 Middle lobe collapse. There is increased density in the right mid-zone (blue) with loss of definition of the right heart border. The right hemidiaphragm is still clearly seen. The position of the horizontal fissure in a normal lung is shown with a white dotted line (1); however, in this case the horizontal fissure has been pulled downwards (2). The volume loss from the collapsed middle lobe has slightly pulled the trachea to the right side (3).

Right lower lobe collapse

The right lower lobe collapses inferiorly and medially.

Features of right lower lobe collapse on a chest radiograph: Figure 7.12

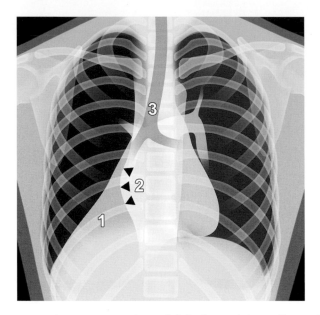

Figure 7.12 Diagrammatic representation of right lower lobe collapse. Triangular shaped increased opacity at the right lung base medially (1), loss of the right hemi-diaphragm silhouette, right heart border still visible (2), tracheal deviation to the right (3).

- Triangular opacification at the right base medially.
- Loss of definition of the right hemidiaphragm.
- Elevation of right hemidiaphragm (pulled up by collapsed lobe).
- Depression of right hilum (pulled down by collapsed lobe).
- **The right heart border is not obscured.**
- The remainder of the right lung looks blacker than the left lung (the right upper lobe and middle lobe over-inflate to compensate for the reduced volume in the hemithorax caused by the collapsed right lower lobe).

Example: Figure 7.13

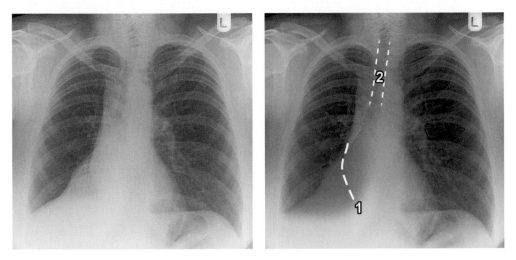

Figure 7.13 Right lower lobe collapse. There is a triangular opacity at the right base medially (blue) with loss of definition of the right hemidiaphragm. The right heart border (1) is still clearly seen. The volume loss from the collapsed right lower lobe has slightly pulled the trachea to the right side (2).

Left upper lobe collapse

The left upper lobe collapses inwards (medially), upwards and anteriorly.

Features of left upper lobe collapse on a chest radiograph: Figure 7.14

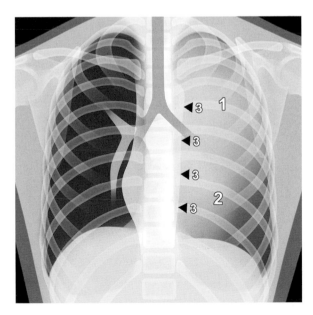

Figure 7.14 Diagrammatic representation of left upper lobe collapse. Increased density in the left hemithorax with a 'veil-like' appearance (1), loss of the left heart border (2), outline of the descending thoracic aorta remains visible (3).

- Increased density in the left upper and mid zones.
- **'Veil-like' opacification in the left hemithorax with no clear lower border.**
- Loss of definition of left upper cardiac border and left mediastinal margin.
- The descending thoracic aorta remains visible (outlined by air in the adjacent left lower lobe).
- Elevation of left hilum (pulled up by collapsed lobe) and left hemidiaphragm.
- Trachea may be deviated to the left (collapsed lobe pulls trachea).

Example: Figure 7.15

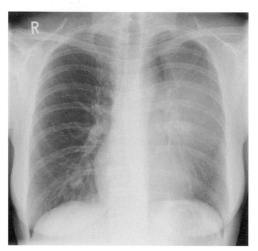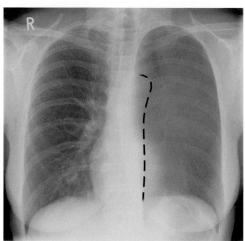

Figure 7.15 Left upper lobe collapse. There is increased density in the left upper and mid zones with no clear inferior border and a loss of definition of the left heart border. You can, however, see the outline of the left hemidiaphragm and descending thoracic aorta (black dotted line) as there is still air in the left lower lobe, which lies adjacent to these structures.

Left lower lobe collapse

The left lower lobe collapses inferiorly and medially.

Features of left lower lobe collapse on a chest radiograph: Figure 7.16

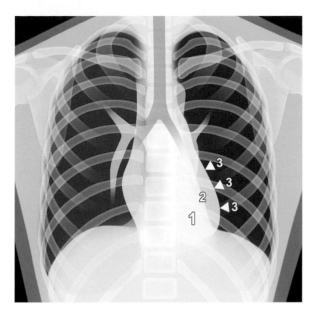

Figure 7.16 Diagrammatic representation of left lower lobe collapse. Triangular shaped increased opacity at the left lung base medially (1), loss of definition of the medial part of the left hemidiaphragm, outline of collapsed left lower lobe (2), left heart border still visible (3).

- Triangular opacification overlying the left heart medially (giving so called **'double heart border'** sign).
- Loss of definition of the medial aspect of the left hemidiaphragm.
- Elevation of the left hemidiaphragm (pulled up by collapsed lobe).
- Depression of left hilum (pulled down by collapsed lobe).
- **The left heart border is not obscured.**
- The remainder of the left lung looks blacker than the right lung (the left upper lobe over-inflates to compensate for the reduced volume in the hemithorax caused by the collapsed left lower lobe).

Example: Figure 7.17

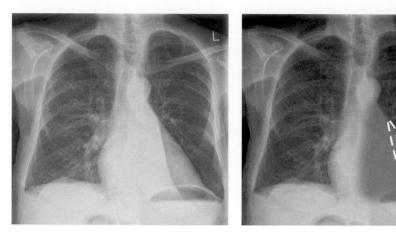

Figure 7.17 Left lower lobe collapse. There is a triangular opacity projected over the left side of the heart (blue). The lateral margin of the collapsed left lower lobe (1) together with the left heart border (2) can both be seen separately giving the 'double heart border' sign. There is elevation of the left hemidiaphragm (normally it should lie lower than the right) and reduced density of the rest of the left lung when compared to the right lung due to left upper lobe hyper-inflation (to compensate for the reduced volume in the left hemithorax caused by the collapsed left lower lobe).

Complete lung collapse

Example 1: Figure 7.18

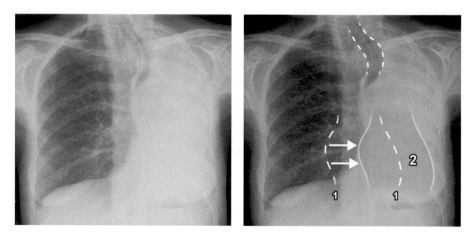

Figure 7.18 Complete left lung collapse. There is increased density throughout the entire left hemithorax and signs of decreased lung volume, such as displacement of the heart/mediastinum towards the collapsed lung and left tracheal deviation. The heart has moved from its normal position (1) to lie in the left hemithorax (2). The trachea is shown in blue and outlined with a white dotted line.

Example 2: Figure 7.19

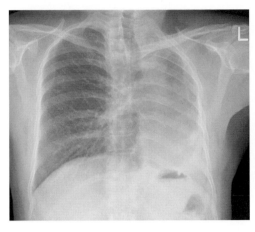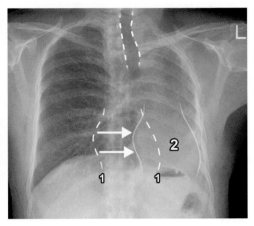

Figure 7.19 Almost complete collapse of the left lung (although there is still a minimal amount of air in the left upper lobe). There is increased density throughout the entire left hemithorax and signs of decreased lung volume, such as displacement of the heart/mediastinum towards the collapsed lung and left tracheal deviation. The heart has moved from its normal position (1) to lie in the left hemithorax (2). The trachea is shown in blue and outlined with a white dotted line.

Pneumonectomy

Pneumonectomy is an **operation to remove a whole lung.** You should know from the patient's clinical history and your clinical examination (scars from previous surgery) that the patient has had a previous pneumonectomy.

Radiological signs of a pneumonectomy

- **Diffuse opacification** and **loss of hemidiaphragm outline** where the lung has been removed.
- **Volume loss in the hemithorax** on the side the lung has been removed and **hyperinflation of the opposite lung field** (appears darker).
- **Mediastinal/tracheal shift** towards the side with no lung.
- You may see **surgical clips** and/or evidence of **rib resection.**

> **Note:** You cannot differentiate between a pneumonectomy and a complete lung collapse on a chest radiograph (unless you can see evidence of a previous thoracotomy) as they may both look the same.

Example 1: Figure 7.20

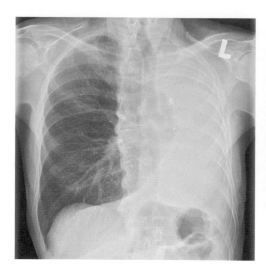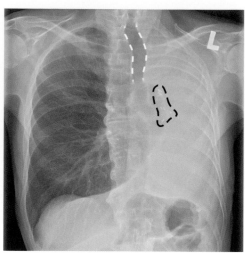

Figure 7.20 Previous left pneumonectomy. There is diffuse opacification throughout the left hemi-thorax (fluid). There is mediastinal shift and tracheal deviation to the left, towards the side of the operation. If you look carefully, you can see surgical clips projected over the left hemithorax (outlined by a blacked dashed line). The trachea is marked in blue and outlined with a white dotted line.

Immediately after a pneumonectomy operation, the hemithorax is filled with a mixture of air and fluid giving the appearance of a hydropneumothorax. You may see surgical staples, clips, evidence of a thoracotomy (part of the rib missing), or subcutaneous emphysema from the recent surgery. After a while, the air is absorbed by the body and replaced with fluid, giving a whiteout of the hemithorax. The sequence of events after a pneumonectomy is shown on the following page (*see* Figure 7.21).

Example 2: Figure 7.21

Figure 7.21 Serial radiographs of the same patient.

1. **Pre-operative radiograph** showing a mass lesion (red) in the right hilar region. The patient subsequently underwent a right pneumonectomy.
2. **One-week post-operative radiograph** showing evidence of a recent right pneumonectomy. There is diffuse opacification (fluid, green) in the inferior two thirds and air (pneumothorax, blue) in the superior third of the right hemithorax. You can see a horizontal air–fluid level (A) where the debris/fluid meets the air. There is a line of staples from the recent surgery. (B). There is also subcutaneous emphysema (yellow) and a small left-sided pleural effusion (green).
3. **One-month post-operative radiograph** showing diffuse opacification throughout the right hemithorax (fluid) and tracheal deviation to the right (blue), towards the side of the operation.

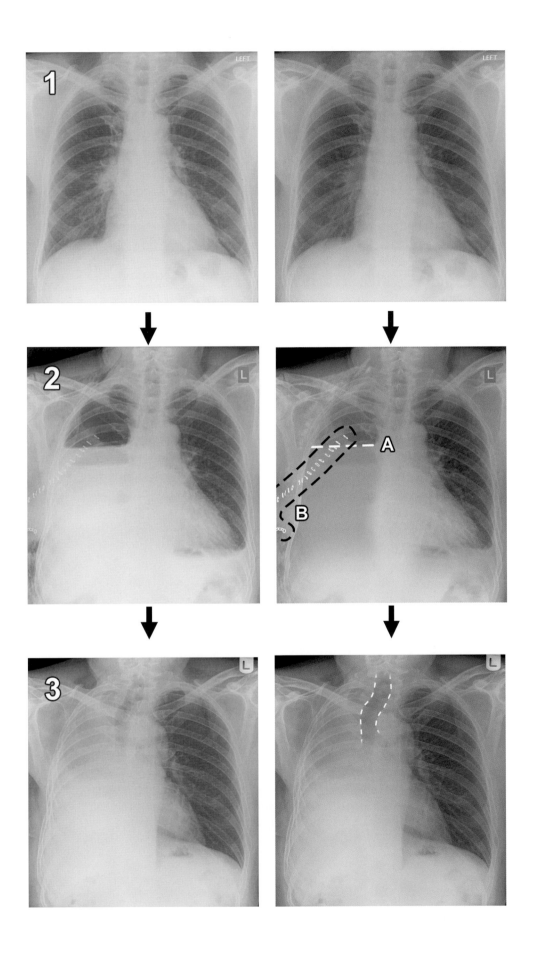

Solitary mass lesion

A solitary mass lesion is a term used to describe a **discrete area** of **whiteness** situated within a lung field. It is not necessarily circular (it can be round, oval, or irregular). The main worry is that it could be a malignancy.

Radiological factors to assess

- **Size** – greater than 1 cm in diameter is more concerning.
- **Margin** – irregular, lobulated, or spiculated margin suggests malignancy.
- **Cavitation** (*see* p. 48) – both neoplasm and infection may cause cavitation.
- **Calcification** – would appear dense white (like bone). Rare in malignancy. More commonly seen in benign lesions.
- **Compare with a previous CXR** – to assess growth.
- **If you see one, look carefully for other mass lesions.**

Differential diagnosis

1. **Neoplasm.**
   a. **Primary lung malignancy:**
      - Evidence of rapid growth in a short time (multiple examinations).
      - Irregular, lobulated, or spiculated margin.
      - No calcification.
   b. **Solitary metastasis:**
      - Look for evidence of previous mastectomy – can give clue as to possible cause, e.g. breast cancer.
2. **Benign mass lesion.**
   a. **Intrapulmonary,** e.g. hamartoma (often contain calcium) and benign lung cysts.
   b. **Extrapulmonary,** e.g. neurofibromata.
3. **Infection.**
   a. **Tuberculosis (TB).**
      i. **Primary TB:**
         - Peripheral lung mass/consolidation (Ghon focus).
         - Associated with enlarged hilar lymph nodes.
      ii. **Tuberculoma** (remnants of previous TB infection):
         - Calcification common.
         - Well-defined margin.
         - Around 2 cm diameter.
         - Unchanged on serial CXR examinations.
   b. **Other infection.**
      - Localised area of consolidation or abscess.
4. **Arteriovenous malformations.**
   - Feeding arteries and draining veins may be seen.

Example 1: Figure 7.22

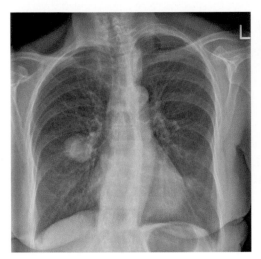
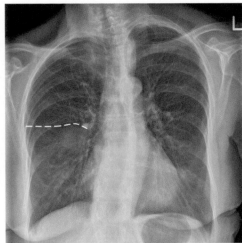

Figure 7.22 Large mass lesion (red) in the middle lobe. You know it is located within the middle lobe because if you look carefully you can see that the mass is pushing up the horizontal fissure (white dashed line), which separates the right upper lobe and middle lobe.

Example 2: Figure 7.23

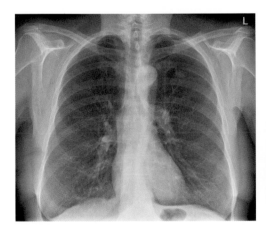
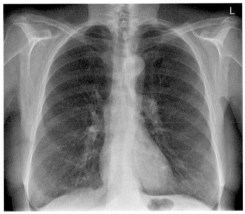

Figure 7.23 Small solitary mass lesion (red) in the left upper zone.

Example: Figure 7.38

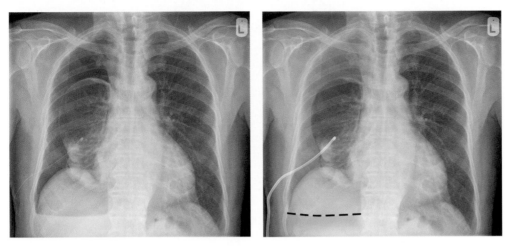

Figure 7.38 Right-sided hydropneumothorax. You can see a horizontal air–fluid level (black dashed line) between the pneumothorax (blue) above and pleural fluid (green) below. There is also a chest drain in situ (white).

Pleural effusion

A pleural effusion is the **accumulation of fluid** in the **pleural cavity** (the space between the parietal and visceral layers of the pleura) (Figures 7.39 and 7.40).

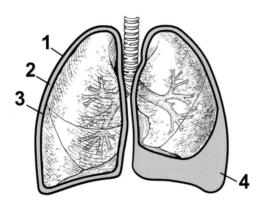

Figure 7.39 Diagrammatic representation of a left-sided pleural effusion. The fluid in the pleural space is shown in green. In a normal 70 kg male the intrapleural space contains only a few millilitres of pleural fluid. Parietal pleura (1), pleural space (2), visceral pleural (3), pleural effusion (4).

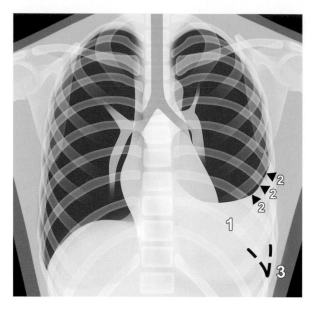

Figure 7.40 Diagrammatic representation of a left-sided pleural effusion. There is a homogenous dense opacity (1) with a concave upper margin giving a typical 'meniscus shape' (2) and loss of visualisation of the left costophrenic angle (3).

This may be caused by the following.

- **Transudate** (<30 g/l of protein):
    - heart failure (congestive heart failure, pericardial effusion)
    - liver failure (cirrhosis)
    - renal failure
    - protein loss (nephrotic syndrome)
    - reduced protein intake (malnutrition)
    - iatrogenic (peritoneal dialysis).
- **Exudate** (>30 g/l of protein):
    - infection (pneumonia, TB)
    - infarction (pulmonary emboli)
    - malignancy (primary lung malignancy, mesothelioma, metastasis)
    - collagen vascular disease (rheumatoid arthritis, systemic lupus erythematosus)
    - pancreatitis (usually left-sided effusion)
    - trauma/surgery (associated with rib fractures).

The radiograph appearances do not change with the nature of the fluid; therefore, transudate, exudate, blood (haemothorax), pus, or lymph (chylothorax) all look the same. Fluid appears white and on an erect chest radiograph the patient is upright so the fluid from a pleural effusion drains to the bottom of the chest.

> **Note:** Collapse may also cause whiteness at the base of a lung. To help differentiate between collapse and a pleural effusion, look at the trachea. With collapse, there is a loss of lung volume and the trachea is deviated towards the affected side. With an effusion, the trachea is usually central (or if massive, may even be pushed towards the opposite side).

Classical radiological appearance of a pleural effusion

- Homogenous dense opacity (homogenous whiteness).
- Loss of the costophrenic angle.
- Meniscus (i.e. higher laterally than medially); therefore, the upper margin will be concave.
- Loss of hemidiaphragm.
- No air bronchogram.

Example 1: Figure 7.41

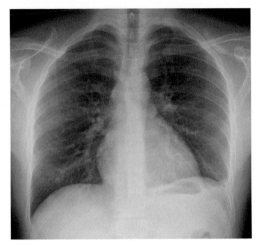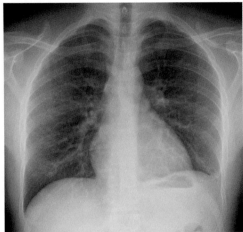

Figure 7.41 Small left-sided pleural effusion (green). There is loss of visualisation of the left costophrenic angle. The upper edge is concave in shape giving a 'meniscus' appearance laterally.

Example 2: Figure 7.42

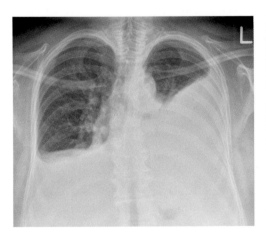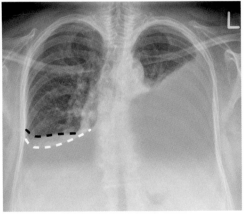

Figure 7.42 Bilateral pleural effusions (green). The effusions are homogenous, dense opacities and the left-sided effusion is larger than the right. There is a loss of visualisation of the left and right costophrenic angles and both hemidiaphragms. The upper edges are concave in shape giving a 'meniscus' appearance laterally. The right-sided effusion appears to have two upper edges; one is fluid tracking anterior to the lung and the other is fluid tracking posteriorly (white and black dashed lines).

Example 3: Figure 7.43

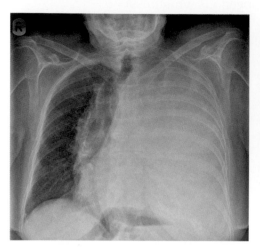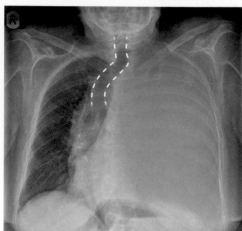

Figure 7.43 Massive left-sided pleural effusion (green). There is a homogenous, dense opacity in the left hemithorax with loss of visualisation of the left costophrenic angle and left hemidiaphragm. There is no meniscus as the pleural effusion extends all the way to the apex of the left lung. You can tell that this is a pleural effusion and not lung collapse or a pneumonectomy because there is mass effect, i.e. the trachea (outlined with a white dotted line and shown in blue) and mediastinum are pushed away from the increased density.

Note: Massive pleural effusions such as the one in the example above are frequently associated with an underlying mass lesion. If there is a history of trauma, also consider a haemothorax or chylothorax.

Notes on haemothorax: A haemothorax looks the same as a pleural effusion on a chest radiograph. The cause of a haemothorax is usually traumatic: a blunt or penetrating injury to the thorax results in **rupture of the parietal or visceral pleura.** This rupture allows blood to spill into the pleural space, equalising the pressures between the pleural space and the lungs.

Blood loss into this space may be massive as each hemithorax can hold **30–40%** of a person's blood volume.

Other than trauma, a haemothorax may occur as a complication of:

- **pneumothorax**
- **pulmonary infarct**
- **anticoagulant therapy,** which may potentiate the ability of a chest injury to cause a haemothorax.

Pulmonary oedema

Pulmonary oedema is **fluid accumulation in the lungs** that causes flooding of the alveoli with fluid. This causes severe disturbance of gas exchange across the alveolar surface and can lead to respiratory failure.

Note: Pulmonary oedema differs from a pleural effusion because in pulmonary oedema the fluid is in the alveoli and in a pleural effusion the fluid is in the pleural space.

Causes of pulmonary oedema

1. **Cardiogenic pulmonary oedema:**
   - **Heart failure.** Failure of the heart to remove fluid from the pulmonary circulation (left ventricular dysfunction or mitral valve disease).
2. **Non-cardiogenic pulmonary oedema:**
   - **Renal failure** with fluid overload.
   - **Iatrogenic** fluid overload.
   - **Adult respiratory distress syndrome (ARDS).**

Radiological appearances

- **Symmetrical, diffuse 'fuzzy' opacification** (with sparing of the peripheries): especially in the mid- and lower zones where the pulmonary venous pressure is highest due to gravity (provided the patient is upright).
- **Upper lobe vascular prominence:** vessels in the upper lobe are larger than vessels in lower lobe on erect chest radiograph (due to increased pulmonary vascular resistance in the lower zones).
- **Peri-bronchial opacification:** the bronchi are thickened when viewed end-on. This is a radiographic sign occurring when excess fluid builds up in the small airways causing localised patches of atelectasis (lung collapse). This causes the area around the bronchus to appear more prominent on a radiograph.
- **Peri-hilar haziness:** hazy opacification around the hilar regions.
- **Septal lines** (*see* p. 64).
- In acute cases you may see the characteristic **'bat's wing' pattern.**

Bat's wing' pattern opacification

In acute pulmonary oedema you may see the radiological appearance of bilateral or unilateral **ill-defined opacification** confined to the **central (peri-hilar) area** of the lungs, **extending laterally to stop 2–3 cm before the periphery of the lung.**

- The opacity takes the shape of a bat's wing (you may have to use your imagination here!).
- To date there is no explanation for this distribution of disease, which occurs almost exclusively in patients with pulmonary oedema.
- Classically associated with left ventricular failure and resultant pulmonary oedema.

Example 1: Figure 7.44

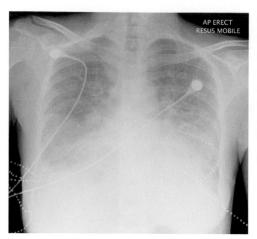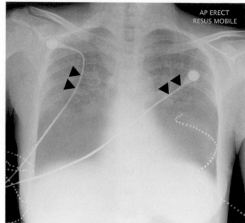

Figure 7.44 Pulmonary oedema (pink) seen as symmetrical, diffuse 'fuzzy' opacification in the mid and lower zones. You can also see small bilateral pleural effusions (with blunting of the costophrenic angles), two ECG leads (black arrowheads), and clothing artefacts (dotted lines).

Example 2: Figure 7.45

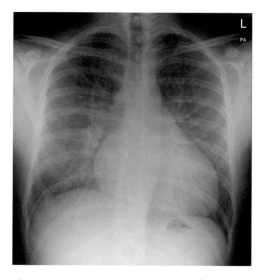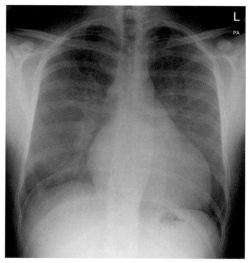

Figure 7.45 Pulmonary oedema (pink) seen as symmetrical, diffuse 'fuzzy' opacification particularly in the mid-zone and peri-hilar region. You can also see cardiomegaly.

Example 3: Figure 7.46

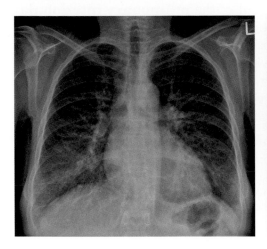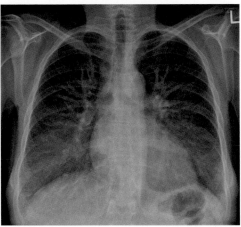

Figure 7.46 Pulmonary oedema (pink). There is bilateral diffuse 'fuzzy' opacification in the mid and lower zones. There is evidence of upper lobe vascular prominence (red) as vessels in the upper zone appear slightly larger than usual. There are also a few septal lines which are seen best in the right lower zone.

Example 4: Figure 7.47

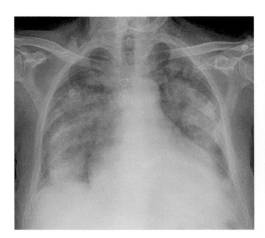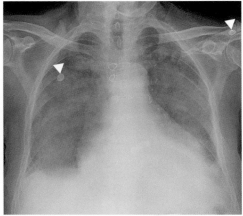

Figure 7.47 Pulmonary oedema with the 'bat's wing' pattern (pink). There is ill-defined opacification bilaterally extending laterally to stop 2–3 cm before the periphery of the lung. You can also see cardiomegaly, median sternotomy wires projected over the midline, and, if you look carefully, there are several tiny clips projected over the left side of the heart/mediastinum. The clips and sternotomy wires are from a previous coronary artery bypass graft (CABG). Two ECG stickers are also noted (white arrowheads).

Septal lines

Septal lines are caused by **engorgement** of the **pulmonary interlobular septal lymphatics** by fluid, tumour, or fibrosis.

Septal lines are found around the periphery of the lungs, extending inwards from the pleural surface. They are invisible on the normal chest radiograph. They become visible when thickened by fluid, tumour, or fibrosis.

On a chest radiograph, the lines are **very fine** and seen around the **peripheries** at a **90° angle** to the pleura. They are easy to miss so *actively* look for them.

> **Note:** Originally described by Kerley, septal lines are traditionally known as **Kerley 'A' lines** (in the central portion of the lung) or **Kerley 'B' lines** (in the periphery of the lung). They should now be collectively referred to as **'septal lines'**.

Causes of septal lines

- **Interstitial pulmonary oedema** (e.g. from pulmonary venous hypertension secondary to heart failure).
- **Lymphangitis carcinomatosa.** In advanced malignancy, the septal lymphatics may become obstructed or infiltrated by tumours leading to the appearance of septal lines. They are usually bilateral and may be associated with hilar node enlargement.
- **Fibrosis in pneumoconiosis** (very rarely).

Example: Figure 7.48

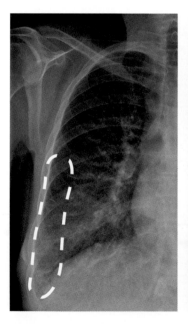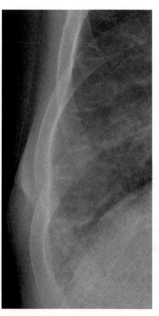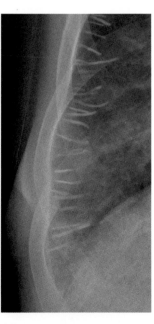

Figure 7.48 Septal lines (yellow). The left image shows the peripheral location of septal lines (white dashed lines). The middle and right image show a magnified view of the septal lines which are typically very fine and seen around the peripheries at a 90° angle to the chest wall.

Asbestos-related lung disease

Inhalation of **asbestos fibres** is an industrial hazard that can lead to chest disease. Patients may be entitled to compensation as it is considered to be an occupational lung disease. The incidence of primary lung malignancy in people who have worked with asbestos is five times higher in non-smokers and 50 times higher in smokers.

There are three disease categories:

1. **benign pleural disease**
2. **asbestosis**
3. **mesothelioma.**

Benign pleural disease

The distinctive radiological features are **asbestos plaques.** Asbestos plaques are **pleural plaques – areas of pleural thickening** caused by **asbestos fibres.** They usually contain calcification and give a localised area of whiteness on a chest radiograph. Patients may also develop small pleural effusions.

Radiological features

- **Pleural plaques** are seen on a chest radiograph as they contain calcification. They appear as *irregular opacities* with *well-defined edges.* They are usually *bilateral.* Often, they are also seen running *along the diaphragm.*
- **Diffuse pleural thickening** which appears as a thickened line around the periphery of the lung.
- **Pleural effusions** may develop after a latent period averaging 10 years after exposure.

> **Note:** Compare to a previous radiograph. Pleural plaques are slow growing and will probably be visible on an old radiograph.

Example of pleural plaques: Figure 7.49

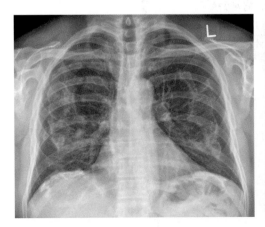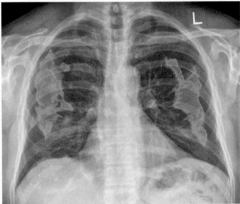

Figure 7.49 Pleural plaques in both lungs (green). Note the well-defined edges and calcification (whiteness) within. There are also calcified pleural plaques running along the diaphragm.

Asbestosis

Asbestosis is the term for the **interstitial fibrosis** that develops in approximately 50% of patients with industrial asbestos exposure. It is a **chronic inflammatory condition** affecting the **interstitial tissue** of the lungs, occurring after long-term, heavy exposure to asbestos (e.g. mining).

Radiological features

- **Fibrosis** with some **volume loss** (*see* Fibrosis, p. 50 for examples).
- **Calcified pleural plaques.**

Mesothelioma

A mesothelioma is a **malignant tumour** that develops in the **pleura,** usually unilaterally and causes pleuritic type chest pain (Figure 7.50 and 7.51): **5–10%** of asbestos workers develop malignant mesothelioma. It has a **latent period of 20–45 years.**

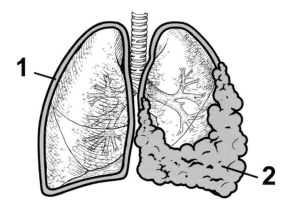

Figure 7.50 Diagrammatic representation of a left-sided mesothelioma. The pleural space is shown in green and you can see that the mesothelioma easily spreads within the pleural space encasing the lung. Pleural space (1), mesothelioma (2).

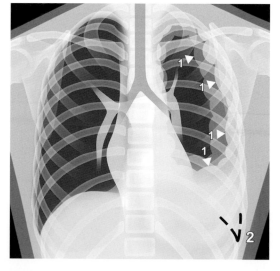

Figure 7.51 Diagrammatic representation of a left-sided mesothelioma. There is peripheral lobular opacification (1) surrounding the left lung and loss of visualisation of the left costophrenic angle (2).

On a chest radiograph it gives characteristic **pleural opacification** (from diffuse, progressive thickening of the pleura and associated malignant pleural effusion) and evidence of **chest wall invasion** (metastasis).

Radiological features

- The **edges** of the opacification are **lobular** in nature *(suggests malignancy)*.
  - Look at the upper edges of the opacification. There should be **no meniscus** *(this is because the main differential diagnosis to rule out is a pleural effusion).*
- There may be **loss of lung volume** on the affected side (*increases suspicion of mesothelioma*).
- Evidence of chest wall invasion (**rib destruction** or **soft tissue mass in the chest wall**) may be the only feature to differentiate mesothelioma from benign disease.

Note: Pleural tumours could be due to mesothelioma, other secondaries, benign tumours (rare), or pleural sarcoma (very rare).

Example 1: Figure 7.52

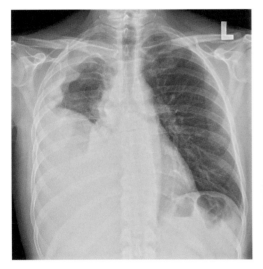
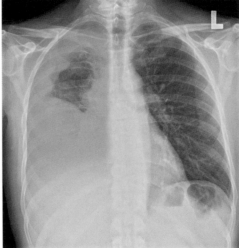

Figure 7.52 Large right-sided malignant mesothelioma (green). Note that the whiteness surrounding the whole right thoracic cavity is lobular in nature and is not constrained to a particular lung lobe.

Example 2: Figure 7.53

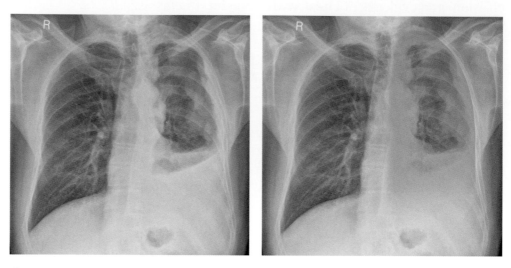

Figure 7.53 Large left-sided malignant mesothelioma (green). Note that the whiteness surrounding the whole right thoracic cavity is lobular in nature and is not constrained to a particular lung lobe. There is also an associated left pleural effusion.

8

C – Circulation

How to review the heart and mediastinum

- Look at the heart size. The width of the heart should be no more than half the total width of the thorax.
- Look at the great vessels (pulmonary vessels and aorta).

The Latin for heart is 'cor' (as in cor pulmonale); therefore, remember to look at the 'core' of the X-ray, i.e.:

- Look at the mediastinum, both hila, and look for a hiatus hernia.

What to look for

Dextrocardia

Dextrocardia literally means that the heart is arranged in a **perfect mirror image** to the normal positioning. Therefore, the heart is in the **right hemithorax,** with the **cardiac apex directed to the right.** Basically, the heart is the wrong way around.

In some patients, all the visceral organs are mirrored (heart, lungs, liver, spleen, etc.) and are arranged in the exact opposite position. This is called **situs inversus totalis.** In situs inversus totalis the heart and two-lobed lung are both on the right and the three-lobed lung is on the left. As this arrangement is a perfect mirror image, the relationship between the organs has not changed.

Chest X-rays for Medical Students: CXRs Made Easy, Second Edition.
Christopher Clarke and Anthony Dux.
© 2020 John Wiley & Sons Ltd. Published 2020 by John Wiley & Sons Ltd.
Companion website: www.wiley.com/go/clarke-cxr-2e

As the organs below the hemidiaphragm are also on the opposite side, you may see the gas in the stomach beneath the right hemidiaphragm, rather than beneath the left hemidiaphragm.

You must be cautious when diagnosing dextrocardia using a chest radiograph. More commonly the image may have been 'flipped' during processing or the image markers may have been placed the wrong way around. If there is any doubt as to the diagnosis, have a low threshold for repeating the radiograph, just to be sure.

> **Note:** ECG leads and defibrillation pads must be placed in reversed positions on a person with dextrocardia.

Example: Figure 8.1

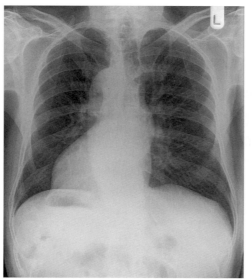 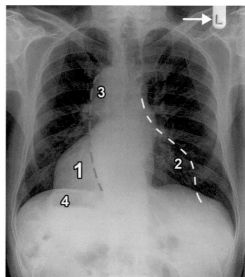

Figure 8.1 Dextrocardia. The heart is in the right hemithorax with its apex directed to the right (1) as opposed to the standard position (shown with a white dashed line, 2). The thoracic aorta is also on the opposite side to normal (green dashed line, 3). Also, you can see gas within the stomach (blue, 4) beneath the right hemidiaphragm rather than beneath the left hemidiaphragm. This indicates that the abdominal organs are also on the opposite side, so this patient has situs inversus totalis.

Cardiomegaly (enlarged heart)

If the width of the heart is **more than half the total width of the thorax,** the patient has cardiomegaly. The width should be measured horizontally and is the longest possible distance between the left and right heart borders.

> **Note:** You can only comment on the cardiac size on a PA (posterior–anterior) chest radiograph. This is because on AP (antero–posterior) or supine radiographs the mediastinum and cardiac size will appear wider due to venous distension and magnification (see p. 7). Therefore, you should not comment on the cardiac or mediastinal size on an AP/supine radiograph.

Example: Figure 8.2

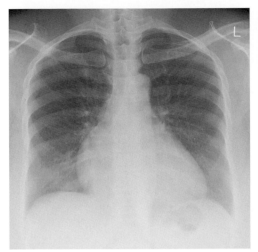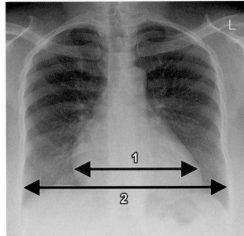

Figure 8.2 A PA chest radiograph showing cardiomegaly. The shorter red arrow (1) marks the width of the heart. The longer black arrow (2) marks the width of the thoracic cavity. As you can see, the width of the heart is greater than half the width of the thoracic cavity; therefore, the heart is enlarged (cardiomegaly). You can also see median sternotomy wires from previous surgery.

Normally two-thirds of the heart should lie to the left of the midline and one-third to the right of the midline. The left ventricle forms the left heart border and the right atrium forms the right heart border. Both the left atrium and right ventricle outline are not visible on a normal chest radiograph. This is because the right ventricle lies anteriorly, and the left atrium lies posteriorly; therefore, they have no definable border on a frontal chest radiograph.

The image of the heart that you see on the PA chest radiograph comprises mainly of the **left ventricle,** therefore cardiomegaly is usually due to **left ventricle enlargement.** The most common reason for the heart to be enlarged is **heart failure,** so look for signs of left ventricular failure on the rest of the radiograph (*see* Heart failure, p. 105).

Left atrial enlargement

The left atrium may be seen on a PA chest radiograph as enlargement of the **left atrial appendage (Figure 8.3).** The left atrial appendage is normally concave in shape, but if the left atrium is enlarged (usually secondary to **mitral stenosis**) there is a **loss of concavity and straightening of the left atrial appendage.** Sometimes, atrial enlargement is so great that the left atrial appendage bulges outwards.

Radiological signs of left atrial enlargement

- Straightening or bulging of the left atrial appendage.
- Widening of the carinal angle (*see* p. 25).
- The right heart border appears further to the right side than usual.
- You may see a 'double shadow' at the right heart border due to the outline of the enlarged left atrium.

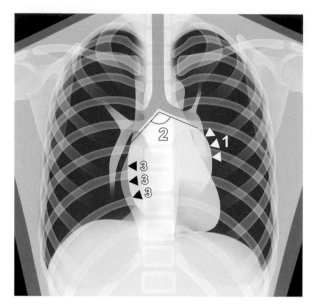

Figure 8.3 Diagrammatic representation of left atrial enlargement. Bulging of the left atrial appendage (1), widening of the carinal angle (2), 'double shadow' at the right heart border (3).

Example: Figure 8.4

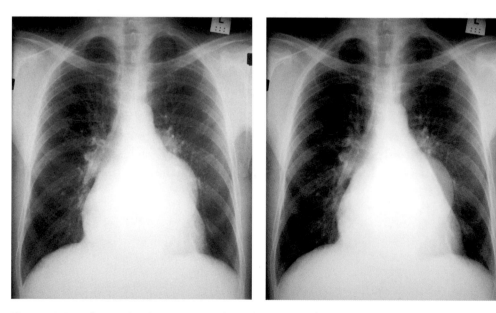

Figure 8.4 Left atrial enlargement. The left atrial appendage is bulging out (orange) and the right heart border appears further over to the right than usual. In this case, the left atrium is enlarged secondary to mitral valve disease.

Widened mediastinum

The mediastinum is the **central part of the thorax.** It contains the heart, the great vessels, oesophagus, trachea, phrenic nerve, vagus nerve, sympathetic chain, thoracic duct, thymus, and central lymph nodes (including hilar lymph nodes). If you think the mediastinum is wider than normal, relate this finding to the patient's clinical history. **Hilar enlargement also gives a widened mediastinum** and is covered in a separate section on p. 76.

Note: Always check to ensure the radiograph is not rotated. A rotated radiograph can make the mediastinum look falsely widened.

Important causes of a widened mediastinum:

- aortic dilatation (aortic aneurysm or aortic dissection);
- lymph node enlargement;
- dilatation of the oesophagus;
- oesophagectomy with subsequent gastric pull-up or colonic interposition;
- thyroid enlargement;
- thymic tumour.

The level of the widening (upper, central, lower) can help determine the cause.

- Upper mediastinal widening: more likely to be paratracheal lymphadenopathy, thyroid or thymus in origin.
- Central or lower mediastinal widening: more likely to be hilar enlargement, aortic widening, lymphadenopathy, dilatation of the oesophagus, or a thymic tumour.

Specific radiological signs to look for

- **If you suspect widening of the aorta:**
    - follow its outline. You may see a continuous edge that widens to form the edge of the enlarged mediastinum;
    - look for calcification in the wall of the aorta and if you can see a line of calcium, follow it:
        - if the calcified aortic wall bulges, there is likely to be an aortic aneurysm;
        - if the line of calcium separates from the edge of the aortic outline, then this would be in keeping with an aortic dissection.

Note: The aorta may become tortuous in the elderly and this may mimic a widened aorta. Some radiologists describe this as 'unfolding of the aorta'.

- **If you suspect an enlarged thyroid:**
    - look at the position of the trachea. An enlarged thyroid will displace or narrow the trachea.

Example 1: Figure 8.5

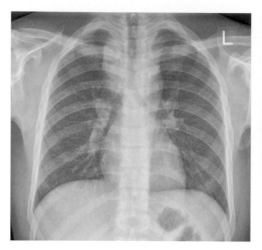
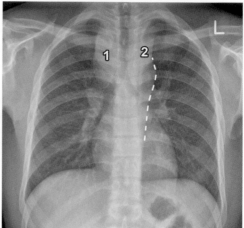

Figure 8.5 Right (1) and left (2) paratracheal lymph node enlargement (orange). The upper mediastinum appears widened with a smooth lobular appearance. The outline of the descending thoracic aorta is marked with a white dotted line. Do not confuse the descending thoracic aorta with lymph node enlargement. You can tell it is the aorta as the outline continues inferiorly down the length of the thorax.

Example 2: Figure 8.6

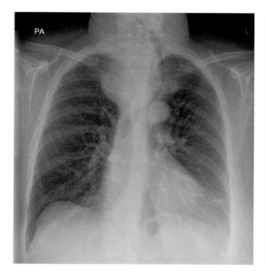
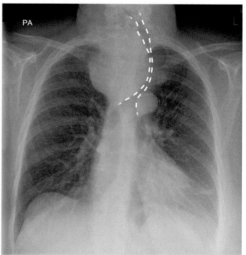

Figure 8.6 Large upper mediastinal mass (orange) causing narrowing and displacement of the trachea (blue and outlined with a white dotted line) to the left. Subsequent imaging with a CT scan of the chest confirmed a large multinodular thyroid goitre.

Example 3 – A patient with central chest pain radiating to the back: Figure 8.7

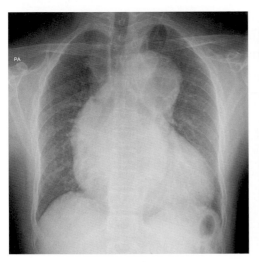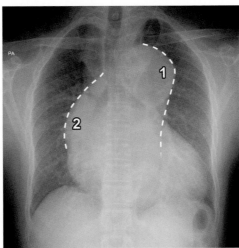

Figure 8.7 Widened mediastinum due to enlargement of the thoracic aorta (orange). The outline of the descending thoracic aorta is marked with a white dotted line (1). The outline of the ascending thoracic aorta (normally not clearly seen) is marked with a white dotted line (2). A CT scan of the chest was performed which showed a large aortic dissection.

Example 4 – A patient with a history of lower oesophageal cancer: Figure 8.8

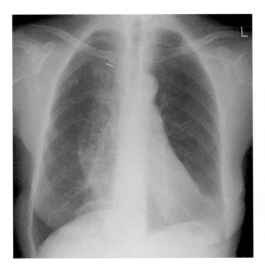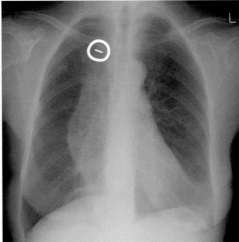

Figure 8.8 Widened mediastinum due to gastric pull-up (orange). This patient had a previous Ivor Lewis oesophagectomy for oesophageal cancer. The oesophagus was resected and the stomach was 'pulled-up' into the chest to act as a conduit to replace the resected oesophagus. The stomach is much wider than the oesophagus, therefore the gastric pull-up causes widening of the mediastinum on a chest radiograph. There is also a surgical clip (white circle) projected over the right upper zone, likely from the previous surgery.

Hilar enlargement

Suspect hilar enlargement if:

- one hilum is **bigger** than the other;
- one hilum is **denser** than the other;
- there is **loss of the normal concave shape** (this may be the first sign of hilar enlargement.
- Location of the hilar regions on a normal radiograph (Figure 8.9).

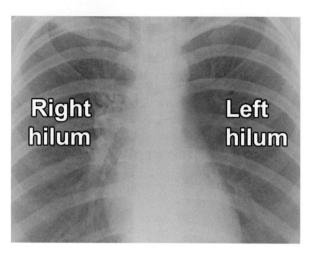

Figure 8.9 Right and left hila regions marked in blue.

Each hilar region consists of the:

1. **pulmonary artery**
2. **bronchus**
3. **lymph nodes** (not visible unless enlarged)
4. **superior and inferior pulmonary veins.**

In assessing hilar enlargement, you must decide which of these structures are involved. Hilar enlargement always requires further investigation, usually with a CT chest initially.

The three causes of unilateral hilar enlargement

1. **Unilateral enlargement of the hilar lymph nodes (lymphadenopathy):**
   - Smooth lobular appearance.
   - May have calcium deposits (very bright white).
   - Look at the periphery for lung lesions (tumour, TB).
   - Look at the rest of the mediastinum. Malignant hilar enlargement may be associated with superior mediastinal lymphadenopathy.
   - Causes include: infection (e.g. TB), spread from primary lung tumour, primary lymphoma, or sarcoidosis (rarely unilateral).

2. **Central bronchial carcinoma superimposed over the hilar region:**
   - Spiculated, irregular, or indistinct margins.
   - Look at the periphery for other lung lesions or bony lesions (metastases).
   - Look at the rest of the mediastinum. Malignant hilar enlargement may be associated with superior mediastinal lymphadenopathy.
3. **Enlarged vasculature:**
   - If the branching pulmonary arteries appear to arise from an apparent mass, this would indicate an enlarged main pulmonary artery.
   - Vascular margins are usually smooth.
   - Causes include: pulmonary artery aneurysm or post-stenotic dilatation of the pulmonary artery.

The two causes of bilateral hilar enlargement

1. **Pulmonary hypertension:**
   - Pulmonary arterial enlargement is a cause of bilateral hilar enlargement. If the branching pulmonary arteries appear to arise from an apparent mass, this would indicate an enlarged main pulmonary artery.
   - May be associated with reduction in the peripheral vascularity. The edges of the lung fields are often darker than usual and the central area often whiter (this is often associated with congenital heart disease).
   - Look for a cause, e.g. signs of mitral stenosis or features of chronic lung disease.
   - Causes include: obstructive lung disease (e.g. asthma, COPD), left heart disease (e.g. mitral stenosis, LVF), left to right shunts (e.g. ASD, VSD), recurrent pulmonary emboli, or primary pulmonary hypertension.
2. **Bilateral enlargement of the hilar lymph nodes (lymphadenopathy)**
   - Same appearance and causes as for unilateral hilar lymph node enlargement, except now seen on both sides! Lymphoma and sarcoidosis are more likely.

Example: Figure 8.10

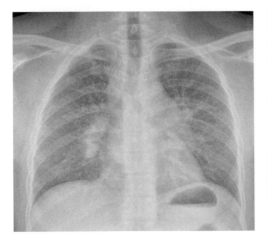 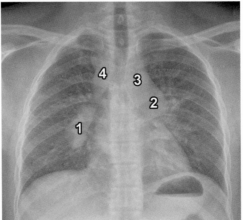

Figure 8.10 Bilateral hilar and paratracheal lymph node enlargement (orange). There is increased density and widening of the mediastinum due to enlarged right hila lymph nodes (1), enlarged left hila lymph nodes (2), enlarged left paratracheal lymph nodes (3), and enlarged right paratracheal lymph nodes (4).

Hiatus hernia

A hiatus hernia is the **herniation of the stomach into the thorax.** On an erect chest radiograph, it appears as a 'mass' behind the heart with an **air–fluid level.**

Example 1: Figure 8.11

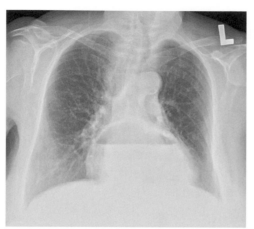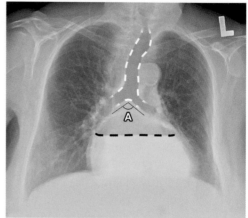

Figure 8.11 Very large hiatus hernia seen projected over the heart. There is an air–fluid level (black dashed line) between the gastric contents (yellow) and gastric air bubble (blue). The hiatus hernia is so large that is it causing widening of the carinal angle (A). The trachea is shown in blue and outlined with a white dotted line.

Example 2: Figure 8.12

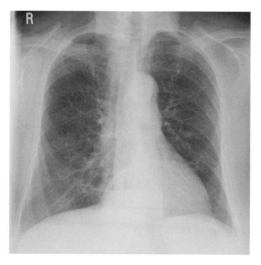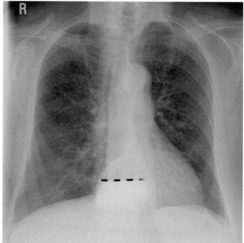

Figure 8.12 Hiatus hernia seen projected over the heart. There is an air-fluid level (black dashed line) between the gastric contents (yellow) and gastric air bubble (blue).

9 D – Disability

How to review the bones

- Look for a **fracture** or **abnormality** of the **ribs.**

> **Tip:** Try rotating the radiograph 90° (Figure 9.1). When you look at a radiograph normally, your eyes are trained to look at the anatomy of the lungs and heart. However, rotating the image tricks your brain and your eyes tend to focus on the dense parts (ribs and other bones) making it easier to spot a fracture.

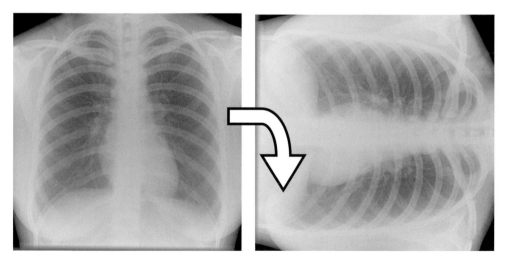

Figure 9.1 Rotating the radiograph makes it easier to appreciate the ribs and look for fractures or bony abnormalities (this is a normal chest radiograph).

Chest X-rays for Medical Students: CXRs Made Easy, Second Edition.
Christopher Clarke and Anthony Dux.
© 2020 John Wiley & Sons Ltd. Published 2020 by John Wiley & Sons Ltd.
Companion website: www.wiley.com/go/clarke-cxr-2e

Nasogastric (NG) tube

An NG tube should normally pass through the oesophagus and into the stomach. Look carefully for the correct positioning of an NG tube. A correctly positioned NG tube should:

1. Pass inferiorly in the midline.
2. Cross over the left or right main bronchus (not follow the path of the bronchial tree).
3. Pass below the level of the diaphragm with tip at least 5 cm below the level of the diaphragm.

   Incorrectly positioned tubes can lead to aspiration, pneumonia, and increased morbidity and mortality. If the tip of the NG tube is within the oesophagus, trachea, bronchus, or lung then the tube should be immediately removed and repositioned.

Example of an NG tube in the correct position: Figure 10.7

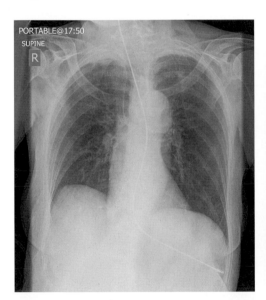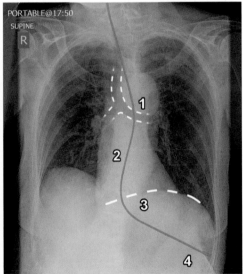

Figure 10.7 Correct positioning of an NG tube (pink). The NG tube is seen crossing the left main bronchus (1) and is projected over the midline (2). It passes inferior to the level of the diaphragm (3) and the tip is projected below the level of the left hemidiaphragm (4). The trachea and left and right main bronchi are outlined with a white dotted line and shown in blue. The left hemidiaphragm is shown with a white dashed line.

Example of an incorrectly placed NG tube: Figure 10.8

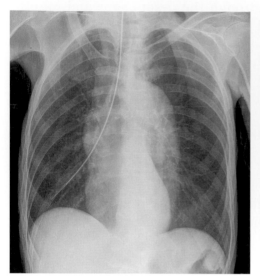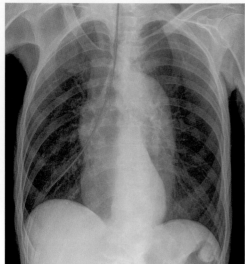

Figure 10.8 Incorrect positioning of an NG tube (pink) which is projected over the right lung. The NG tube has travelled down the trachea, right main bronchus, and intermediate bronchus to end up in either the right lower or middle lobe bronchus. It must be removed immediately and re-inserted.

Example of an incorrectly placed NG tube: Figure 10.9

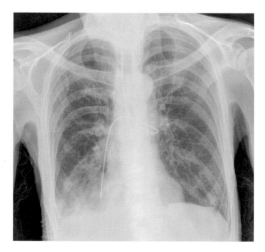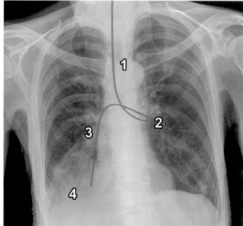

Figure 10.9 Incorrectly positioned NG tube (pink). The NG tube is initially projected over the midline (1); however, rather than crossing the carina, it first passes down the left main bronchus, then loops back on itself (2) and passes down the right main bronchus (3) to end up in the right lung. There is consolidation (green) in the right lower zone, probably due to inappropriate feeding through the NG tube. It must be removed immediately and re-inserted.

Example of an incorrectly placed NG tube: Figure 10.10

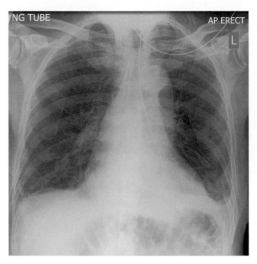
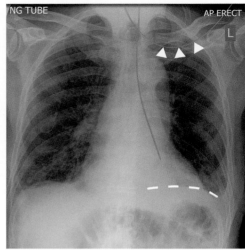

Figure 10.10 Incorrectly positioned NG tube (pink). The NG tube passes to the left side with its tip projected over the left side of the heart. The tube does not pass below the level of the diaphragm (white dashed line) and probably lies within the left lower lobe bronchus. It must be removed immediately and re-inserted. You can also see part of the NG before it enters the nose (white arrowheads) and a small left-sided pleural effusion (green).

Example of an incorrectly placed NG tube: Figure 10.11

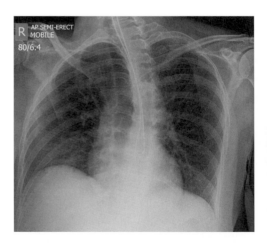
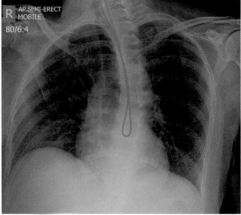

Figure 10.11 Incorrectly positioned NG tube (pink). The NG tube is projected over the midline; however, it is looped in the lower oesophagus with the tip passing superiorly. The tip of the NG tube is not actually visualised on this radiograph, although it is likely to lie in the region of the pharynx. It must be removed immediately and re-inserted.

Vascular access catheters

There are a wide variety of types and location of vascular access catheters; however, the most common type you will come across are central venous catheters which are usually inserted into the left/right internal jugular veins or left/right subclavian veins.

Example of a correctly placed right internal jugular central venous catheter: Figure 10.12

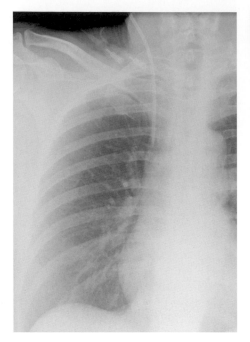
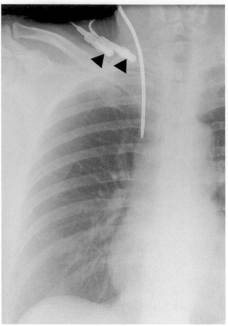

Figure 10.12 Correct positioning of a right internal jugular central venous catheter (white) with tip projected over the superior vena cava. Two caps on the external part of the drain can also be seen (black arrowheads).

Example of an incorrectly placed right internal jugular central venous catheter: Figure 10.13

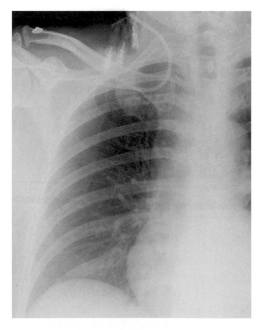
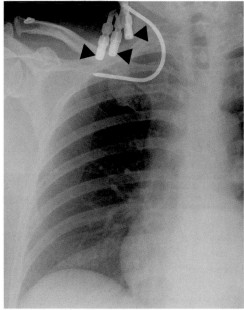

Figure 10.13 Incorrect positioning of a right internal jugular central venous catheter (white). The tip has entered the right subclavian vein rather than the superior vena cava. Three caps on the external part of the drain can also be seen (black arrowheads).

Example of a correctly placed dual-lumen tunnelled central venous catheter: Figure 10.14

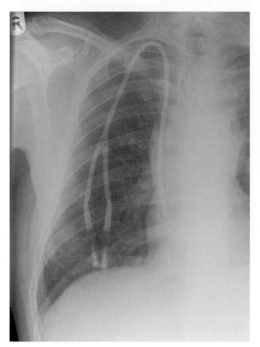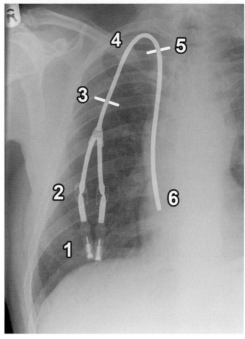

Figure 10.14 Right-sided tunnelled dual-lumen central venous catheter (white). You can see two caps (1) at the end of each lumen and two plastic clamps (2) pinching the lumen. The line then enters the patient's skin (approximately position 3, white line), curves through the subcutaneous tissue (4), and enters the right internal jugular vein (approximately position 5, white line) to pass into the right brachiocephalic vein and superior vena cava. The tip (6) is just within the right atrium.

Peripherally inserted central catheter (PICC or PIC line)

A PICC is a form of intravenous access that enters a peripheral vein (normally in the arm) and extends to the superior vena cava. It often stays in place for days or weeks.

Example of a correctly placed PICC: Figure 10.15

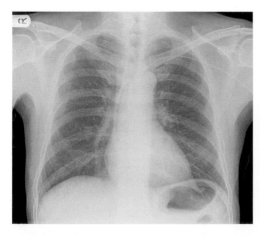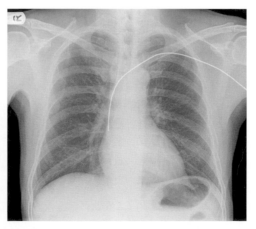

Figure 10.15 Normal position of a left-sided peripherally inserted central catheter (white). The catheter should follow the course of the axillary vein, subclavian vein, and brachiocephalic vein with its tip (often very difficult to appreciate on a plain radiograph) projected over the superior vena cava.

Example of an incorrectly placed PICC: Figure 10.16

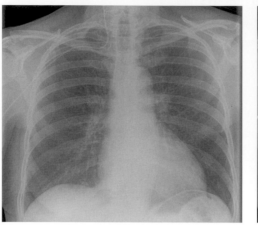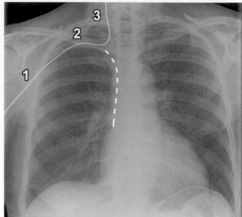

Figure 10.16 Incorrectly positioned right-sided peripherally inserted central catheter (white). The catheter is projected over the right axillary vein (1) and right subclavian vein (2), but then deviates superiorly into the right internal jugular vein (3). The tip is not seen on this radiograph. The line must be re-positioned so that the tip follows the white dashed line to lie in the superior vena cava.

Endotracheal tube (ETT): Figures 10.17 and 10.18

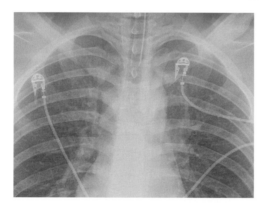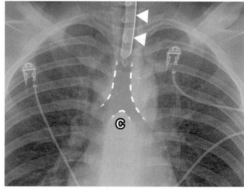

Figure 10.17 Endotracheal tube (white arrowheads) in situ. The tip of the endotracheal tube is situated well above the carina (C) where the trachea (blue) splits into the left and right main bronchi. Two ECG leads are also seen.

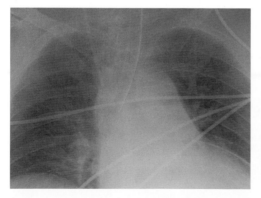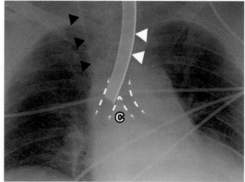

Figure 10.18 Malpositioned endotracheal tube (white arrowheads). The tip of the endotracheal tube is projected over the right main bronchus, below the level of the carina (C). This tube must be withdrawn so that the tip lies above the level of the carina. A right-sided internal jugular central venous catheter (black arrowheads) and multiple ECG leads are also seen.

Tracheostomy tube: Figure 10.19

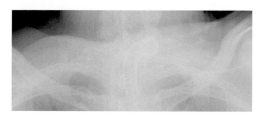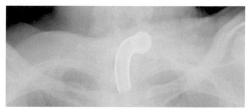

Figure 10.19 Tracheostomy tube (white).

Surgical clips/staples/wires

Surgical clips, staples, and wires are common findings on chest radiographs. It is important to recognise the differences between them.

Example of sternotomy wires: Figure 10.20

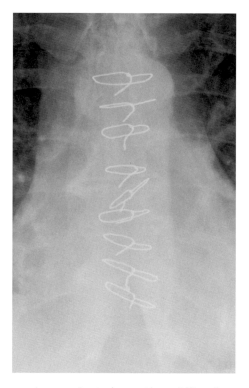

Figure 10.20 Sternotomy wires projected over the midline from a previous median sternotomy.

Example of surgical staples: Figure 10.21

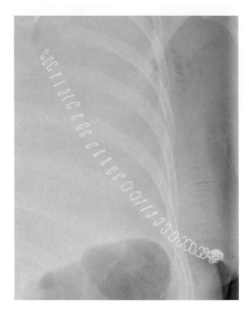

Figure 10.21 Surgical staples from a recent left-sided pneumonectomy.

Examples of surgical clips: Figure 10.22

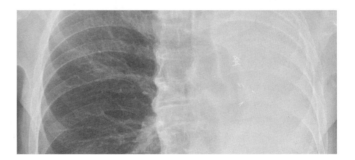

Figure 10.22 Surgical clips projected over the left hemithorax from previous left pneumonectomy.

Examples of artificial heart valves: Figure 10.23

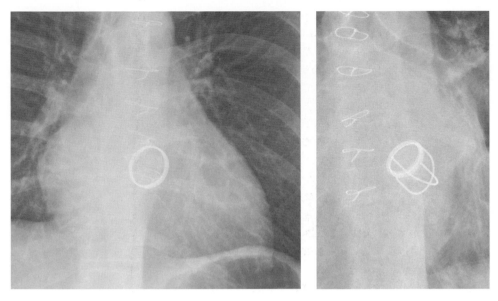

Figure 10.23 Two mechanical heart valves projected over the heart. The valves appear white because they contain metal, absorbing X-rays and appearing radiopaque. In both examples, there are also sternotomy wires from the original operations to insert the heart valves.

Example of a cardiac conduction device: Figure 10.24

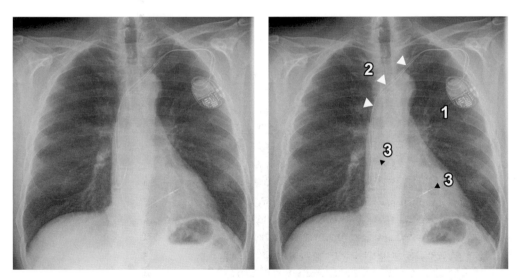

Figure 10.24 Cardiac conduction device (pacemaker). The pulse generator (1) sits within the subcutaneous tissue and, in this example, it is projected over the left pectoral region – although the location can vary. This device has two leads (white arrowheads, 2) which extend from the pulse generator into the heart (tips shown with black arrowheads, 3). Devices come in various shapes and sizes and may have one, two, three, or more leads.

Example of ECG leads and loop recorder device: Figure 10.25

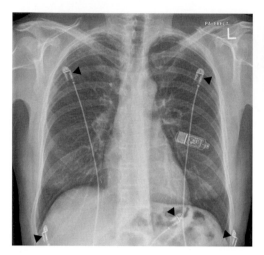
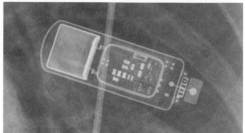

Figure 10.25 Five ECG leads (black arrowheads) and a loop recorder (zoomed image) which has been placed subcutaneously in the anterior chest wall. This device may pick up arrhythmias when they occur and is subsequently interrogated by an external reading device.

Example of breast implants: Figure 10.26

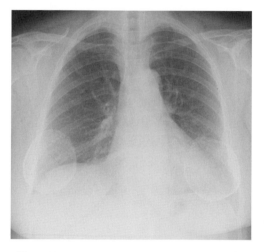
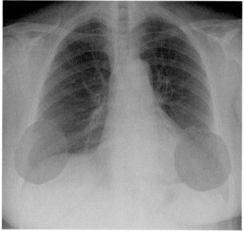

Figure 10.26 Bilateral breast implants (pink).

Nipple markers

Sometimes nipples are seen on a chest radiograph as two rounded opacities. Unfortunately, these can sometimes be mistaken for lung nodules! If there is uncertainty, radiologists can mark the nipples and repeat the X-ray. If the opacities are seen within the 'nipple markers' then this confirms that they are in fact just nipples and there is nothing to worry about.

Example: Figure 10.27

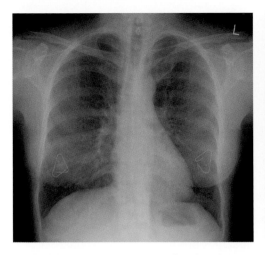
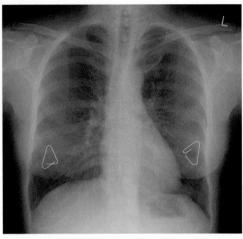

Figure 10.27 Two opacities (red) projected over the lower zones. The radiologist was not sure whether these represented nipples or lung nodules, so taped nipple markers (in this case paper clips) to both nipples. The repeat radiograph (shown here) clearly shows that both opacities are within the nipple markers, confirming these to be the patient's nipples rather than lung nodules.

Foreign bodies

Key points to keep in mind:

- Artefacts projected over the chest may actually be outside of the body (e.g. metal on clothing or items in pockets).
- Following facial trauma, look carefully for an aspirated tooth. It will appear as a small triangular/rectangular shaped opacification and most commonly lodges in one of the main/lobar bronchi.

Example of a coin stuck in the oesophagus: Figure 10.28

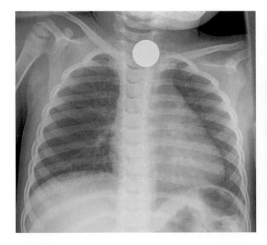
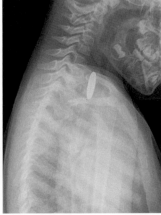

Figure 10.28 A swallowed coin stuck in the oesophagus of a child. The left image shows the AP view and the right image shows a lateral view. This was subsequently removed endoscopically.

Example of shotgun pellets: Figure 10.29

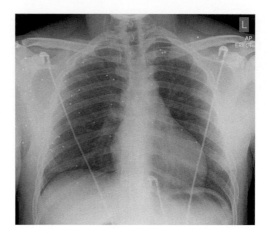

Figure 10.29 Multiple small, round, metallic opacities projected over the chest consistent with shotgun pellets. You can also see three ECG leads.

Example of nipple piercings: Figure 10.30

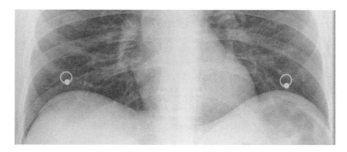

Figure 10.30 Bilateral nipple piercings.

III Common conditions and their radiological signs

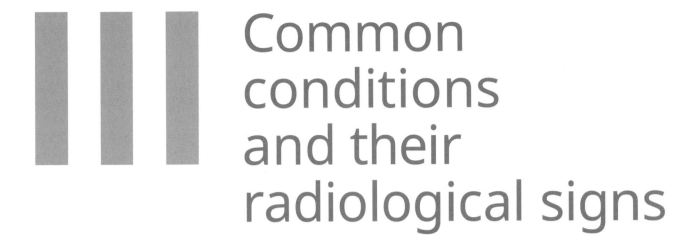

You will come across many of the following conditions in your medical practice; however, not all have distinct features on a chest radiograph. We have mentioned them here to help you understand the role of chest radiographs in the diagnosis and management of these conditions.

Chest X-rays for Medical Students: CXRs Made Easy, Second Edition.
Christopher Clarke and Anthony Dux.
© 2020 John Wiley & Sons Ltd. Published 2020 by John Wiley & Sons Ltd.
Companion website: www.wiley.com/go/clarke-cxr-2e

11

Common conditions and their radiological signs

Pulmonary embolism (PE)

There are no specific radiological features of pulmonary embolism (PE) on a chest radiograph and although some associated features are described – e.g. hilar enlargement (caused by thrombus), pulmonary infarction (wedge shaped consolidation at the periphery of the lung), focal atelectasis, and localised oligaemia – these findings are inconsistently present and very non-specific, thus a positive diagnosis of PE cannot be made with a chest radiograph.

The purpose of a chest radiograph in suspected PE is to look for other conditions that mimic PE in their clinical presentation; for example, a pneumothorax or consolidation.

The current 'Gold Standard' for the diagnosis of pulmonary embolism is a CT pulmonary angiogram (CTPA).

Primary lung malignancy

The main histological types are non-small cell lung carcinoma (consisting of adenocarcinoma, squamous cell carcinoma, and large cell carcinoma) and small-cell lung carcinoma.

Radiological features

- **Lobulated** or **spiculated mass,** but sometimes with a smooth outline.
- May be **associated with hilar lymph node enlargement, pleural effusion,** and/or areas of **collapse** or **consolidation.**
- **Cavitation found in 15%** (central air lucency, an air–fluid level and a wall of variable thickness). Squamous cell carcinomas frequently cavitate.
- May also see **metastases.**

Chest X-rays for Medical Students: CXRs Made Easy, Second Edition.
Christopher Clarke and Anthony Dux.
© 2020 John Wiley & Sons Ltd. Published 2020 by John Wiley & Sons Ltd.
Companion website: www.wiley.com/go/clarke-cxr-2e

> **Note:** Invasive mucinous adenocarcinoma (a subtype of adenocarcinoma) may have a variable appearance including consolidation, air bronchograms, or widespread pulmonary nodules, rather than as a solitary mass.

Pneumonia

Pneumonia is **inflammation** of the **lung parenchyma** characterised by **filling of the alveoli air spaces** with **exudate** and **inflammatory cells.** On a chest radiograph, pneumonia appears as **consolidation/airspace shadowing**. Pneumonia is usually caused by infection with viruses or bacteria.

> **Note:** Consolidation and pneumonia are not the same thing and the terms should not be used interchangeably. Consolidation refers to any pathological process that involves the replacement of alveolar air by fluid, cells, pus, or other material. That said, pneumonia is by far the most common cause of consolidation.

Types of pneumonia

■ Community-acquired pneumonia ■ Hospital-acquired pneumonia	Bacterial, viral, or fungal infection
■ Aspiration pneumonia	Inhalation of oropharyngeal secretions

Other occasional features of pneumonia on a chest radiograph include:

- air bronchogram
- pleural effusion (parapneumonic effusion)
- cavitation.

It is usual practice in the UK to perform a repeat chest radiograph six weeks following clinical resolution. The purpose of this is to exclude an underlying malignancy which may present as consolidation, or may have been obscured by the consolidation present on the original radiograph.

It is also important to note that a developing pneumonia may not demonstrate consolidation on a chest radiograph initially – this may develop over the course of days. Likewise, consolidation will often persist for a variable period of time once the infectious process has been treated.

Chronic obstructive pulmonary disease (COPD)

Chronic obstructive pulmonary disease (COPD) is a disease of the lungs characterised by long-term breathing problems and poor airflow due to irreversible airway obstruction by chronic bronchitis and/or emphysema. Smoking is the most common cause of COPD and it is a progressive disease, typically worsening over time.

COPD cannot be diagnosed from a chest radiograph. Always confirm COPD from the patient's clinical history and lung function tests.

If COPD is suspected look for the following.

- **Pneumothorax**
    - common in COPD so look for these (they can 'hide' in the lung apices).
- **Mass lesion/metastasis/other signs of lung cancer**
    - a history of smoking is almost universal in COPD so look for evidence of bronchial carcinoma.

Heart failure

Heart failure is a syndrome defined as the **failure of the heart** to **maintain an adequate flow of blood to the tissues.**

There are many different causes of heart failure, but the four main causes are:

1. ischaemic heart disease
2. non-ischaemic dilated cardiomyopathy
3. hypertension
4. valvular heart disease.

Radiological features associated with heart failure

You may see a combination of one or more of the following five main features of heart failure on a chest radiograph. These are shown in Figure 11.1.

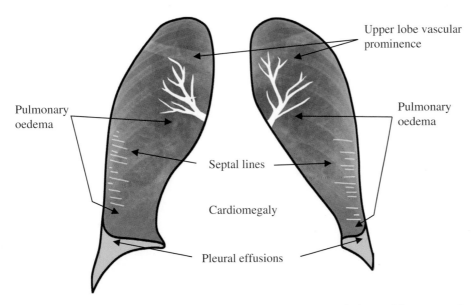

Figure 11.1 Diagrammatic representation of the potential radiological features of heart failure.

1. **Cardiomegaly.**
2. **Pulmonary oedema** (pink):
    - +/- the atypical **'bat's wing' pattern shadowing**.
3. **Upper lobe vascular prominence** (white):
    - vessels in upper lobes appear larger than vessels in the lower lobes on an erect chest radiograph due to increased pulmonary vascular resistance in the lower zones due to dependent oedema.

4. **Septal lines** (light grey):
   - due to fluid in the pulmonary lymphatics.
5. **Pleural effusions** (green):
   - fluid leaks from the vessels into the pleural space.

Example: Figure 11.2

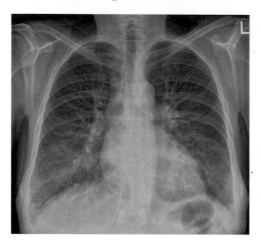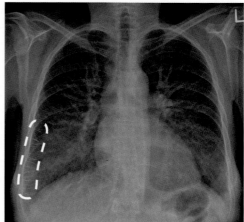

Figure 11.2 A patient with heart failure. There is bilateral diffuse 'fuzzy' opacification in the mid and lower zones in keeping with pulmonary oedema (pink). There is evidence of upper lobe vascular prominence (red) as vessels in the upper zone appear slightly larger than usual. There are also septal lines which are seen best in the right lower zone (yellow, surrounded by white dashed lines). This patient does not happen to have pleural effusions and the heart is not enlarged (although it is at the upper limit of normal).

Tuberculosis

Tuberculosis (TB) is an infection most often caused by *Mycobacterium tuberculosis,* affecting mainly the respiratory tract, though it can involve any system in the body. Patients prone to infection are those who are immunosuppressed, those who are homeless, and those from countries or areas with a high incidence.

Tuberculosis has various manifestations in the lung and often presents in the lung **apices.** There is a lot of crossover between the radiological appearances of primary TB (initial infection), secondary TB (reactivation of previous infection), and previous (old) TB infection. Radiological appearances commonly associated with the different stages of TB are listed below.

Radiological features to look for

- **Primary TB:**
  - peripheral lung mass/consolidation (Ghon focus);
  - enlarged hilar lymph nodes.
- **Secondary TB** (also known as **post-primary** or **reactive TB**):
  - consolidation often with cavitation;
  - typically in upper lobes or apical segments of the lower lobes;
  - may be associated with pleural effusions and/or pleural thickening.

- **Previous (old) TB** (as healing progresses, features you may recognise are):
  - fibrosis and volume loss;
  - calcified foci;
  - pleural calcification;
  - **tuberculoma.** ◄──── *A tuberculoma is a localised granuloma with a well-defined margin, often containing calcification. They are roughly 2 cm in diameter and remain unchanged on serial chest radiograph examinations.*
- **Miliary TB:**
  - discrete 1–2 mm nodules distributed evenly throughout the lung fields due to haematogenous spread.

Example 1: Figure 11.3

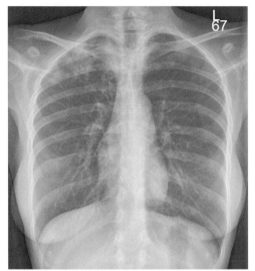
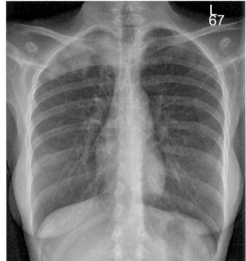

Figure 11.3 Primary TB with right apical consolidation (green). There is patchy opacification at the apex of the right lung.

Example 2: Figure 11.4

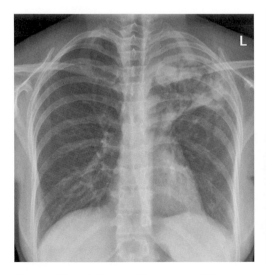
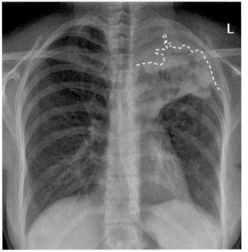

Figure 11.4 Primary TB at the left lung apex. There is pleural thickening at the left apex seen as a homogenous opacification extending inwards from the edge of the thoracic cavity – this is likely to be reactive from the TB. There is also left upper lobe patchy consolidation with some volume loss and reticulonodular opacification suggestive of fibrotic change. The pleural thickening is marked in green superiorly and the consolidation/fibrosis is marked in green inferiorly. A dotted white line separates the pleural thickening (above) from the consolidation/fibrosis (below).

Example 3: Figure 11.5

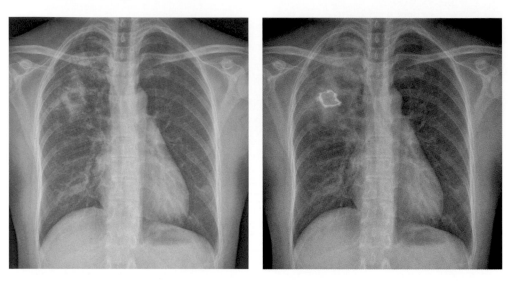

Figure 11.5 Primary TB with patchy right upper lobe consolidation (green) and cavity formation (yellow). The wall of the cavity is shown in light yellow.

Example 4: Figure 11.6

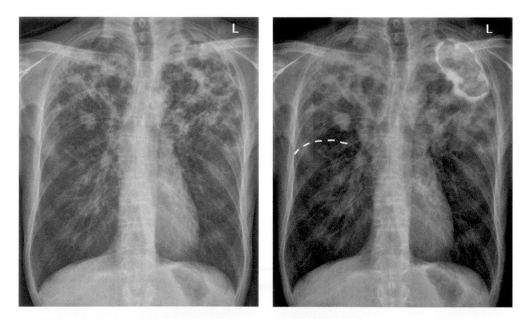

Figure 11.6 Primary TB with bilateral upper lobe consolidation (green) and cavity formation (yellow). There is patchy opacification in both upper lobes. We know this is primarily consolidation rather than fibrosis as there is no significant volume loss. If you look closely, you can see that the horizontal fissure (white dashed line) is not deviated upwards. The wall of the cavity is shown in light yellow.

Example 5: Figure 11.7

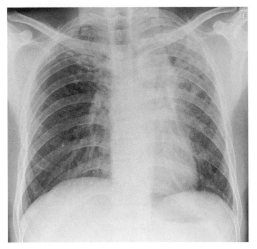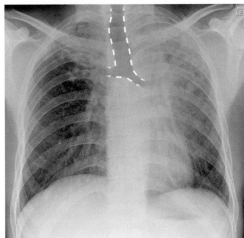

Figure 11.7 Secondary TB (reactivation) with bilateral upper lobe volume loss, left upper zone consolidation (green), left hilar lymph node enlargement (orange), and old TB changes in the right upper lobe (green). There is patchy opacification in both upper lobes. There is elevation of both hila with the left and right main bronchi pulled superiorly causing widening of the carinal angle. The trachea and both main bronchi are outlined with a white dotted line and shown in blue.

Example 6: Figure 11.8

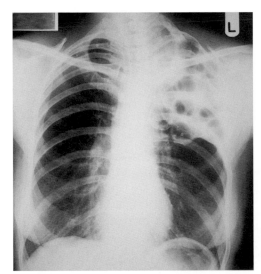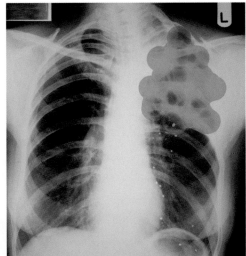

Figure 11.8 Old (previous) TB in a patient who had a thoracoplasty and plombage due to previous TB infection. Plombage was a surgical method used before the introduction of TB antibiotics to treat TB of the upper lobe of the lung. The term derives from the French word 'plomb' (lead) and refers to the insertion of an inert substance into the pleural space, the theory being that if the diseased lobe of the lung was physically forced to collapse, it would heal more quickly. You can see the plombage (purple) in the left upper zone and also some calcified foci (yellow) in the left lung.

Examples 7, 8, and 9: Figure 11.9

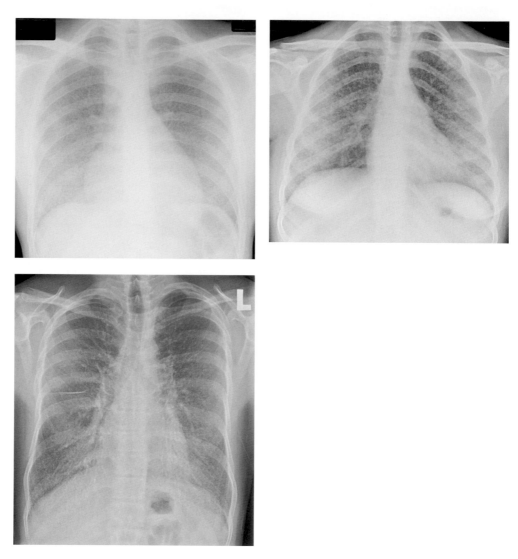

Figure 11.9 Three different chest radiographs of patients with military TB throughout both lungs. There are discrete 1–2 mm nodules distributed evenly throughout the lung fields.

Glossary

Abscess   a localised collection of pus surrounded by inflamed tissue.

Aetiology   the cause of a disease.

Air bronchogram   the radiographic appearance of an air-filled bronchus that is surrounded by fluid-filled or solid alveoli.

Alveoli   tiny air sacs within the lungs where the exchange of oxygen and carbon dioxide takes place.

Anterior   located in front of or towards the front of a structure.

Anticoagulant   a substance that prevents the clotting of blood.

AP (anteriorposterior)   the X-ray tube is placed in front of the patient and the X-rays pass in the anteriorposterior direction.

Apex (of the lung)   meaning the tip of something, it refers to the most superior portion of the lung (*pleural:* **apices**).

Arteriovenous malformation   an abnormal connection between veins and arteries, usually congenital.

Asbestos plaques   deposits of fibrous tissue that develop in the pleura as a result of asbestos exposure.

Asbestosis   an irreversible chronic inflammatory condition affecting the parenchymal tissue of the lungs caused by the inhalation and retention of asbestos fibres. It is one of the causes of lung fibrosis.

Ascending   moving towards a higher level or position.

Aspirate   to suction or to inhale, e.g. fluid into the lungs after vomiting.

Atelectasis   collapse of lung tissue affecting part or all of one lung.

Attenuated   having undergone a process of attenuation (*see* **Attenuation**).

Attenuation   the process by which a beam of radiation is reduced in energy when passing through some material.

Auscultation   the act of listening for sounds made by internal organs, such as the heart and lungs, to aid in the diagnosis of certain disorders, usually using a stethoscope.

Axilla   analogous to the armpit (*pleural:* **axillae**).

'Bat's wing' pattern   the radiological appearance of bilateral or unilateral ill-defined opacities confined to the central (peri-hilar) area of the lungs, as seen in acute pulmonary oedema.

Benign   not recurrent or progressive; not malignant.

Bifurcation   where a structure splits or divides into two.

Bilateral   involving both sides.

Biochemistry   the laboratory department studying the chemical composition of a biological substance, e.g. protein content in a pleural fluid aspirate.

Bronchial   relating to the bronchi (*see* **Bronchus**).

Chest X-rays for Medical Students: CXRs Made Easy, Second Edition.
Christopher Clarke and Anthony Dux.
© 2020 John Wiley & Sons Ltd. Published 2020 by John Wiley & Sons Ltd.
Companion website: www.wiley.com/go/clarke-cxr-2e

Bronchial breathing breath sounds of a harsh or blowing quality, heard on auscultation of the chest, made by air moving in the large bronchi.

Bronchiectasis a persistent or progressive lung condition characterised by dilated thick-walled bronchi.

Bronchogram *see* **Air bronchogram.**

Bronchoscopy a technique for visualising the inside of the airways using a bronchoscope.

Bronchus a subdivision of the trachea serving to convey air to and from the lungs (*pleural:* **bronchi**).

Calcification the process by which calcium builds up in soft tissues.

Cannula a hollow tube that is inserted into a body cavity, duct, or vessel to drain or administer a substance.

Carcinoma a malignant tumour derived from epithelial tissue.

Cardiomegaly enlargement of the heart. If the width of the heart on a PA chest radiograph is more than half the total width of the thorax, then the patient has cardiomegaly.

Cardiomyopathy a disease or disorder of the heart muscle.

Carina the site of tracheal bifurcation.

Carinal angle the angle between the left and right mainstem bronchi.

Cavitation a hole in the lung with a wall, lumen, and contents.

Chronic obstructive pulmonary disease (COPD) an umbrella term for the condition affecting people with chronic bronchitis, emphysema, or both.

Collapse *see* **Atelectasis.**

Computed tomography (CT) a medical imaging technique that uses X-rays to produce an image of a detailed cross-section of tissue.

Computed tomography pulmonary angiography (CTPA) a diagnostic test using computed tomography (CT) to obtain an image of the pulmonary arteries. Its main use is to diagnose a pulmonary embolism (PE).

Concave curving inwards.

Concavity *see* **Concave.**

Connective tissue stroma; a fibrous tissue of mesodermal origin supporting organs, filling the spaces between them, and forming tendons and ligaments.

Consolidation also known as airspace opacification, is the replacement of alveolar air by fluid, cells, pus, or other material.

Contrast the difference in absorption between one tissue and another.

COPD *see* **Chronic obstructive pulmonary disease.**

Costophrenic angle the angle between the ribs and the diaphragm on a chest radiograph.

Crepitation a crackling sound made by tissue, caused by the presence of gas.

CT *see* **Computed tomography.**

CTPA *see* **Computed tomography pulmonary angiography.**

CXR abbreviation for chest X-ray.

Cytology the laboratory department studying cells, e.g. cell numbers and types in a pleural fluid aspirate.

Density the mass per unit volume.

Dependent oedema an abnormal accumulation of fluid in the intercellular spaces of the body that appears to be influenced by gravity.

Diaphragm the musculomembranous partition separating the thoracic and abdominal cavities and acting as the major muscle for inspiration.

Diverticulum an outpouching of a hollow or fluid-filled viscous, e.g. large bowel diverticulum.

ECG (electrocardiography) a test that records the electrical activity of the heart.

Effusion the escape of fluid into a tissue or cavity (e.g. from blood vessels or lymph into the pleural space).

Electromagnetic radiation a form of energy exhibiting wave-like behaviour as it travels through space. It is classified according to the frequency of its wave.

Electromagnetic spectrum the range of all possible frequencies of electromagnetic radiation.

Emphysema an abnormal distension of body tissues caused by retention of air (*see also* **Chronic obstructive pulmonary disease** *and* **Subcutaneous emphysema**).

Endobronchial within or passing through a bronchus.

Endotracheal within or passing through the trachea.

Engorgement distension of body tissues caused by vascular or lymph congestion.

Erect   upright in position or posture.

Expiration   breathing out.

Exposure   the quantifiable dose of radiation on a subject.

Extrapulmonary   outside of the lungs.

Exudate   an extravascular fluid with high protein content (>30 g/l of protein).

Fibrosis   the formation or development of excess fibrous connective tissue in an organ or tissue as a reparative or reactive process, as opposed to a formation of fibrous tissue as a normal constituent of an organ or tissue (e.g. lung fibrosis).

Fissure   a natural deep cleft separating one lobe from another in the lungs and lined by visceral pleura.

Foreign body   any object originating outside the body.

Ghon focus   an area of granulomatous inflammation in the lung caused by tuberculosis in a previously unaffected individual.

Gland   an aggregation of cells specialised to synthesise a substance for release, such as hormones.

Haemothorax   a condition that results from blood accumulating in the pleural cavity.

Hamartoma   a benign tumour-like malformation resulting from faulty development in an organ and composed of an abnormal mixture of tissue elements that develop and grow at the same rate as normal elements but are not likely to compress adjacent tissue.

Heart failure   an inability of the heart to maintain adequate blood circulation to the peripheral tissues and the lungs.

Hemidiaphragm   half of the diaphragm, the muscle that separates the chest cavity from the abdomen and that serves as the main muscle of respiration.

Hemithorax   one side of the chest.

Hiatus hernia   herniation of the stomach into the thorax.

Hilar   relating to a hilum.

Hilum (of the lung)   the point at which the bronchi, pulmonary arteries and veins, lymphatic vessels, and nerves enter the lung.

Homogenous   uniform in structure or composition throughout.

Horner's syndrome   a clinical syndrome consisting of ipsilateral ptosis, miosis, and anhidrosis caused by damage to the cervical sympathetic nervous system.

Hyperinflation   the lung volume is abnormally increased, with increased filling of the alveoli.

Hypersensitivity pneumonitis   diffuse inflammation of the lung parenchyma and airways caused by hypersensitivity to inhaled organic dusts. One of the causes of lung fibrosis.

Hypertension   high blood pressure.

Hypotension   low blood pressure.

Hypoxia   a pathological condition in which the body or a tissue is deprived of adequate oxygen supply.

Iatrogenic   due to the action of a doctor or a therapy the doctor prescribed.

Idiopathic pulmonary fibrosis   a chronic, progressive form of lung disease characterised by fibrosis of the lungs and where the cause is unknown.

Immunosuppressed   lacking a fully effective immune system.

Infarct   an area of tissue death (necrosis) due to a lack of oxygen, caused by an obstruction of the tissue's blood supply.

Inferior   lower in place or position, the opposite of superior.

Inspiration   breathing in.

Interlobular   between lobules.

Interstitial   relating to the interstitium.

Interstitium   the space between cells in a tissue.

Ionisation   the process in which a neutral atom or molecule gains or loses electrons and thus acquires a negative or positive electrical charge. Ionising radiation produces ionisation in its passage through body tissue or other matter. Ionisation can also cause cell death or mutation (*pleural:* **ionisations**).

IRMER   The Ionising Radiation (Medical Exposure) Regulations. UK legislation laying down the basic measures for radiation protection for patients.

Laparoscopy   a type of minimally invasive surgery in which a small incision (cut) is made in the abdominal wall through which an instrument called a laparoscope is inserted to permit structures within the abdomen and pelvis to be seen.

Laparotomy   a surgical procedure involving a large incision through the abdominal wall to gain access to the abdominal cavity.

Lateral situated at the side; away from the middle; extending away from the median plane of the body.

Left atrial appendage a small out-pouching of the left atrium which, if enlarged, may be seen on a PA chest X-ray.

Lesion a general term referring to almost any abnormality involving any tissue or organ.

Lingula a projection of the left upper lobe that closely opposes the left heart border.

Lobar relating to a lobe.

Lobe a clear anatomical division of the lung that can be determined without the use of a microscope, e.g. the left lung is comprised of two lobes and the right lung is comprised of three lobes.

Lobectomy an operation to remove a lobe of the lung.

Lobular relating to a lobule,

Lobulated made up of lobules.

Lobule in contrast to a lobe, lobules are the lung units distal to a respiratory bronchiole and composed of alveolar ducts, alveolar sacs, and alveoli. They are only visible under a microscope.

Lucency an area that has less density that the surrounding area and as a result appears darker on the radiograph.

Lumen the inner open space or cavity of a tube, e.g. blood vessel, intestine, or a cannula.

Lymph an almost colourless fluid that travels through lymphatic vessels in the lymphatic system and carries cells that help fight infection and disease.

Lymph glands small glands found throughout the body; they are a part of the lymphatic system and play a major role in the immune system.

Lymphadenopathy abnormally enlarged lymph nodes.

Lymphangitis carcinomatosa inflammation of the lymphatics secondary to a malignancy.

Lymphatics small vessels that collect and carry lymph from the body to ultimately drain back into the bloodstream.

Lysis breakdown of a cell.

Magnetic resonance imaging (MRI) a medical imaging technique that does not use ionising radiation, but magnetic fields and radio frequency fields to produce an image of a detailed cross-section of tissue.

Main bronchus one of the two main branches of the trachea. The trachea splits at the carina to give the right main bronchus and left main bronchus.

Malignancy cancerous cells that have the ability to spread to other sites in the body (metastasize) or to invade and destroy tissues.

Medial situated in the middle; extending towards the middle; closer to the middle/median plane of the body.

Median sternotomy wires metal sutures used to close the sternum after a median sternotomy is performed during open heart surgery.

Mediastinal relating to the mediastinum.

Mediastinum the central compartment of the thoracic cavity. It contains the heart, the great vessels, oesophagus, trachea, phrenic nerve, vagus nerve, sympathetic chain, thoracic duct, thymus, and central lymph nodes (including hilar lymph nodes).

Meniscus the concave upper surface of a liquid.

Metastasis the process by which a cancer spreads from the place at which it first arose as a primary tumour to distant locations in the body; the cancer resulting from the spread of the primary tumour.

Metastatic relating to metastasis.

Microbiology the laboratory department studying microorganisms, e.g. the presence and type of bacteria in a pleural fluid aspirate.

Mitotic relating to cell division.

MRI *see* **Magnetic resonance imaging.**

Mucus secretions produced in the bronchial tubes to remove foreign particles from the lung.

Mutation a change in the structure of the genes or chromosomes of an organism.

Nasogastric (NG) referring to the passage from the nose to the stomach.

Nasogastric (NG) tube a tube that is passed through the nose down into the stomach.

Neoplasm an abnormal mass of tissue due to the abnormal proliferation of cells. They may be benign or malignant.

Neurofibroma a tumour, usually benign, that consists of nerve fibres and connective tissue, caused by an abnormal proliferation of Schwann cells (*pleural:* **neurofibromata**).

NG *see* **Nasogastric.**

Nodular opacification small discrete opacities 15 mm in diameter, may be seen on a chest radiograph in patients with fibrosis.

Nuclear medicine the branch or specialty of medicine and medical imaging that uses radionuclides and relies on the process of radioactive decay in the diagnosis and treatment of disease.

Oblique situated in a slanting position.

Oedema *see* **Dependent oedema.**

Oligaemia (pulmonary) deficiency in the volume of blood; reduced circulating intravascular volume.

Opacity an opaque or non-transparent area (*pleural:* **opacities**).

Organogenesis the formation and development or organs.

PA (posterioranterior) the X-ray tube is placed behind the patient and the X-rays pass in the posterioranterior direction.

Pacemaker a small electronic device that is placed in the chest to help control abnormal heart rhythms.

PACS *see* **Picture archiving and communication system.**

Paediatric relating to children.

Pancoast tumour a type of lung cancer defined by its location at the apex of the lung.

Pancoast's syndrome pain and muscle atrophy in the upper limb due to a Pancoast tumour invading the brachial plexus.

Paratracheal adjacent to the trachea.

Parenchyma the functional parts of an organ in the body. This is in contrast to the stroma, which refers to the structural tissue of organs, namely the connective tissues.

Parietal pleura *see* **Pleura.**

PE *see* **Pulmonary embolism.**

Pectoralis major a thick, fan-shaped muscle situated on the anterior chest wall.

Percussion an assessment method in which the surface of the body is struck with the fingertips to obtain sounds that can be heard or vibrations that can be felt.

Peri-bronchial adjacent to the bronchus.

Peri-hilar adjacent to the hilum.

Periphery the outermost boundary of an area; the surface of an object (*pleural:* **peripheries**).

Peritoneal cavity the interior of the peritoneum, the lining of the abdominal cavity.

PET *see* **Positron emission tomography.**

Phrenic nerve the nervous supply to the diaphragm originating from C3-5.

Picture archiving and communication system (PACS) a computer-based digital film storage system for storing X-ray images, thereby eliminating the need for film.

Plaques *see* **Asbestos plaques.**

Pleura a serous membrane that folds back onto itself to form a two-layered membrane structure. The thin space between the two pleural layers is known as the pleural cavity; it normally contains a small amount of pleural fluid. The outer pleura (**parietal pleura**) is attached to the chest wall. The inner pleura (**visceral pleura**) covers the lungs and adjoining structures.

Pleural effusion a condition that results from fluid accumulating in the pleural cavity.

Pleural space (Pleural cavity) *see* **Pleura.**

Pleurisy inflammation of the pleura occurring when an infection or damaging agent irritates the pleural surface. Consequently, the patient may develop sharp chest pains.

Pleuritic pain pain relating to pleurisy.

Pneumoconiosis an occupational lung disease caused by the inhalation of dust, often in mines. One of the causes of lung fibrosis.

Pneumonectomy an operation to remove a lung.

Pneumonia an inflammatory condition of the lung, often due to infection.

Pneumoperitoneum air or gas in the abdominal (peritoneal) cavity.

Pneumothorax a collection of air or gas in the pleural cavity of the chest.

Positron emission tomography a nuclear medicine imaging method similar to computed tomography, except that the image shows the tissue concentration of a positron-emitting radioisotope.

Posterior located behind or towards the rear of a structure.

Projection the X-ray view, i.e. AP, PA, supine, or lateral.

Pulmonary relating to the lungs.

Pulmonary embolism (PE) a blockage of one of the main arteries of the lung or one of its branches by a substance (embolus) that has travelled from elsewhere in the body through the bloodstream (usually a thrombus).

Pulmonary hypertension high blood pressure in the pulmonary arteries that convey blood from the right ventricle to the lungs.

Pulmonary oedema a diffuse extravascular accumulation of fluid in the pulmonary tissues and air spaces due to changes in hydrostatic forces in the capillaries or to increased capillary permeability.

Pus a yellowish-white fluid formed in infected tissue, consisting of white blood cells, cellular debris, and necrotic tissue.

Radiation the transfer of energy in the form of particles or waves.

Radiosensitive sensitive to the biological effects of radiant energy such as X-rays.

Radiotherapy the treatment of disease using radiation directed at the body from an external source or emitted by radioactive materials placed within the body.

Reticular opacification a fine or coarse branching linear pattern produced by thickening of the lung interstitium (connective tissue). The heart loses its normal smooth outline and seems 'shaggy'. It may be seen on a chest radiograph in patients with fibrosis.

Reticulonodular opacification a mixture of reticular-type opacification and nodular-type opacification. Seen on a chest radiograph in patients with fibrosis.

Retroperitoneal situated behind the peritoneum.

Rotation the circular movement of an object around a point or centre of rotation.

Sarcoidosis a disease of unknown origin marked by the formation of granulomatous lesions that may appear in many organs, especially in the liver, lungs, skin and lymph nodes. One of the causes of lung fibrosis.

Sarcoma a malignant tumour derived from connective tissue.

Septal lines the radiographic appearance of engorgement of the pulmonary interlobular septal lymphatics. They are seen around the periphery of the lungs, extending inwards from the pleural surface. They are invisible on the normal chest radiograph and only become visible when thickened by fluid, tumour or fibrosis.

Septum a thin partition or membrane that divides two cavities or soft masses of tissue in an organism.

Shadowing *see* **Opacity.**

Shock a medical emergency in which the organs and tissues of the body are not receiving an adequate flow of blood.

Silhouette an outline that appears dark against a light background or light against a dark background.

SLE *see* **Systemic lupus erythematosus.**

Spiculated spiky.

Spinous process the part of each vertebrae projecting backwards giving attachment to the back muscles.

Squamous cell carcinoma a form of bronchial carcinoma, usually in middle-aged smokers.

Stenotic a structure that is narrowed or strictured.

Sternotomy wires *see* **Median sternotomy wires.**

Subcutaneous just beneath the skin.

Subcutaneous emphysema when air or gas is present in the soft tissue layers under the skin e.g. subcutaneous tissue, muscle, etc.

Subphrenic the area under the diaphragm.

Superior higher in place or position, the opposite of inferior.

Supine lying on the back with face upwards.

Surfactant a substance produced by alveolar cells of the lung to maintain stability of the pulmonary tissue by lowering the surface tension of fluids that coat the lung.

Surgical emphysema *see* **Subcutaneous emphysema.**

Sympathetic chain a paired bundle of nerve fibres that run from the base of the skull to the coccyx.

Systemic lupus erythematosus (SLE) a systemic autoimmune disease that can affect any part of the body. It is one of the causes of lung fibrosis.

Systemic sclerosis a systemic autoimmune connective tissue disease. One of the causes of lung fibrosis.

TB *see* **Tuberculosis.**

Tension pneumothorax a serious type of pneumothorax whereby air enters, but cannot leave, the pleural space. This can lead to a complete collapse of the lung and is a medical emergency. It should be a clinical diagnosis.

Thoracic duct the largest lymphatic vessel in the body, it starts in the abdomen and runs superiorly, ascending the posterior mediastinum before draining into the systemic circulation via the left brachiocephalic vein.

Thoracoplasty a former treatment for pulmonary tuberculosis involving surgical removal of parts of the ribs, thus allowing the chest wall to fall in and collapse the affected lung.

Thoracotomy surgical opening of the chest cavity to inspect or operate on the heart, lungs, or other structures within.

Thorax the chest.

Thymic relating to the thymus.

Thymus a lymphoid organ situated in the centre of the upper chest just behind the sternum.

Thyroid a large endocrine gland situated in the neck.

Tissue an aggregation of similarly specialised cells which together perform certain special functions.

Trachea windpipe.

Transudate an extravascular fluid with low protein content (<30 g/l of protein).

Tuberculoma a tumour-like mass resulting from a localised tuberculosis infection.

Tuberculosis a potentially fatal contagious disease that can affect almost any part of the body but is mainly an infection of the lungs. It is caused by the mycobacterium *Mycobacterium tuberculosis*.

Tumour an abnormal swelling or mass of tissue.

Ultrasound a diagnostic medical imaging technique using ultrasound waves to visualise subcutaneous body structures.

Usual interstitial pneumonitis a form of lung disease characterised by progressive fibrosis of both lungs.

Vagus nerve the 10th cranial nerve, passing through the neck and thorax into the abdomen and supplying sensation to part of the ear, the tongue, the larynx, and the pharynx, motor impulses to the vocal cords, and motor and secretory impulses to the abdominal and thoracic viscera.

Visceral pleura *see* **Pleura.**

Index

Page numbers in *italic* denote figures, and those in **bold** denote glossary entries.
